Facilitating Learning in Practice

Many recent high-profile reports have emphasised the need for improvements and innovations in practice-based education for nursing and midwifery students in the UK to ensure safe care delivery.

Addressing the new NMC standards of proficiency for pre-registration nursing, this book presents five significant areas of practice learning for student nurses and midwives in their pre-registration education and provides a guiding resource for practitioners at a time of significant change in the ethos and structure of practice learning. Each chapter provides a short case study and helpful learning points to assist readers in the application of the themes to their own practice.

This concise and accessible book will act as a key stimulus for reflection on the changes in practice learning environments and will provide invaluable guidance on the new roles of Practice Supervisor, Practice Assessor and Academic Assessor. It will be essential reading for all academics and clinical practitioners who support student nurses and midwives with their practice learning.

Dawn A. Morley is Postdoctoral Research Fellow at Southampton Solent University.

Kathy Wilson is Associate Professor and Head of Practice-based Learning within the School of Health and Education at Middlesex University, London.

Natalie Holbery is Head of Nurse Education, University College London Hospitals (UCLH).

Facilitating Learning in Practice

A Research-based Approach to Challenges and Solutions

Edited by
Dawn A. Morley, Kathy Wilson and Natalie Holbery

Routledge
Taylor & Francis Group

LONDON AND NEW YORK

First published 2019
by Routledge
2 Park Square, Milton Park, Abingdon, Oxon OX14 4RN

and by Routledge
52 Vanderbilt Avenue, New York, NY 10017

Routledge is an imprint of the Taylor & Francis Group, an informa business

British Library Cataloguing in Publication Data
A catalogue record for this book is available from the British Library

Library of Congress Cataloging-in-Publication Data
Names: Morley, Dawn A., editor. | Wilson, Kathy (Associate professor), editor. | Holbery, Natalie, editor.
Title: Facilitating learning in practice : a research-based approach to challenges and solutions / edited by Dawn A. Morley, Kathy Wilson and Natalie Holbery.
Description: Abingdon, Oxon ; New York, NY : Routledge, 2019. | Includes bibliographical references and index.
Identifiers: LCCN 2019005014| ISBN 9781138311763 (hardback) | ISBN 9781138311794 (pbk.) | ISBN 9780429458637 (ebook)
Subjects: | MESH: Preceptorship--methods | Education, Nursing--methods | Midwifery--education
Classification: LCC RT76 | NLM WY 18.5 | DDC 610.73071/1--dc23
LC record available at https://lccn.loc.gov/2019005014

ISBN: 978-1-138-31176-3 (hbk)
ISBN: 978-1-138-31179-4 (pbk)
ISBN: 978-0-429-45863-7 (ebk)

Typeset in Bembo
by Taylor & Francis Books

Contents

Illustrations

Figures

Tables

Introduction: Taking steps towards a new vision of nursing and midwifery practice learning

Dawn A. Morley (morleydawn@yahoo.co.uk), Kathy Wilson and Natalie Holbery

Practice education for nursing and midwifery students in the UK has been a neglected aspect of professional nurse preparation for decades (Morley, Wilson and McDermott, 2017). Following the publication of a series of negative national reports and enquiries on the quality of nurse education (Willis Commission, 2012; Willis, 2015), it seemed that the tide of change had moved towards a systematic review of pre-registration nurse and midwifery provision.

The Nursing and Midwifery Council (NMC), the professions' regulatory body in the UK, led a national consultation to radically change both the structures that supported practice learning and assessment that measures students' clinical progress. In addition to discussions regarding models of support in practice, there is also a clear emphasis on the need for nurses to have the knowledge and skills to undertake more flexible roles and an increasing requirement for these higher order knowledge and skills at the point of registration (NMC, 2017).

Despite the investment from the 1990s to move nurse education into higher education in the UK, there remained a sense that nurse education had fallen short of their original intention to develop 'knowledgeable doers' (UKCC, 1986) in practice. It was speculated that this was the all-important second chance to attain genuine graduate skills for the nursing and midwifery professions (Morley, Wilson and McDermott, 2017). Politically it also fell at a significant time for student presence in higher education. With common university funding arrangements, and the loss of bursaries for nursing students, Draper and Kolyva (2018) argued that nursing and midwifery students could be brought into the agenda of quality processes through the new Office of Students and into a stronger position as consumers.

The new NMC Standards (NMC, 2018) that have resulted encourages a multi-professional and team approach to learning in practice that is in keeping with the model of social and collaborative learning promoted in the book. Sharing responsibility for practice learning amongst all members of the healthcare team offers an opportunity to enhance learner understanding of various roles and perspectives (Leigh and Roberts, 2017), understand the wider system students work in and receive feedback from a range of professionals to inform graduate level practice (Leigh and Roberts, 2018).

A greater emphasis on clinical skills development at undergraduate level is explicit, to prepare the future nursing workforce (NMC, 2018). Changes to the NMC standards are more closely aligned to how other healthcare professions support learning in practice and are designed to encourage tailored, flexible learning for students (Leigh and Roberts, 2018). The Council of Deans of Health (2017a) has also welcomed a focus on leadership skills for the future workforce in the pre-registration nursing standards, emphasising the need for nurses to be strong leaders to navigate the ever changing and complex health care arena (CoDH, 2017b). The book's research makes recommendations, and presents further case studies, on how students' learning could be more individualised with personal relevance to their professional journeys.

Changes to enhance learning in practice to ensure proficient nurses in the future, have also highlighted contentious issues. With the removal of the established mentor role in practice education in the UK there is a significant time implication to develop the existing workforce for student supervision and assessment. The Council of Deans of Health (CoDH, 2017a, p. 17) acknowledge some of the value of separating the roles of the assessor and supervisor but underline the importance of recognising that these changes are to occur in environments 'that operate along traditional lines'. Current staffing shortages could greatly impact on the quality of the student experience. The Royal College of Nursing (RCN, 2017) propose that structured training is needed to develop practice assessors as part of an overall career framework.

As nursing is the largest healthcare profession there is also an issue with preparing other professions to understand the new NMC standards (NMC, 2018) and support the growing number of nursing and midwifery learners in practice. There is agreement by both the RCN (2017) and CoDH (2017a) that interprofessional learning should form an integral part of the nurse education programme creating the potential for enhanced inter-agency working (NHS Employers, 2017) although, again, there are concerns regarding consistency and quality assurance.

The focus on the quality of nurse education has also been matched by a recognised need to increase the nursing workforce leading to the formation of new nursing associate roles in English clinical practice (Draper and Kolyva, 2018). The impact of new roles, working alongside those of preregistration nursing students, has only just begun to be evaluated (Traverse, 2018) but those that facilitate nurse education in practice need to be mindful that this could act as a distraction from the original quality agenda and the potential for investment in preparation of the professional nurse workforce. Certainly, the complexity of the practice environment has been increased by the introduction of new roles and the different emphasis of work-based learning and ways that they are assessed (Draper and Kolyva, 2018). Already early confusion has been highlighted of the nursing associate role in practice against the more established professions (Traverse, 2018). The Health Committee report (2018) on the nursing workforce applauds the development of these new roles to diversify the workforce but cautions that the focus on the development of these new routes has meant that limited attention has been given to retaining the current workforce.

Against this changing practice landscape, this book explores a breadth of research issues pivotal to successful practice learning for nursing and midwifery students and offers an alternative approach to support an inclusive, social model of learning. With the NMC decision to withdraw the established model of clinical supervision through mentorship (CoDH, 2017a) alternative clinical supervision models have presented different approaches on how to support students' learning in practice. This is attracting national interest (Bazian, 2016) and radically different ways of managing student nurses' practice experience are emerging.

In recognition of the proliferation of different models of practice support for students, some areas have appointed clinical coordinators or fellows to evaluate the varying approaches (Baker and Sheehy, 2017). However, evidence suggests that large scale implementation is happening fast with little manoeuvrability for pilot studies and research-based evaluation of those models being implemented. The literature review of Chapters 3, 4 and 5 critique some of the different approaches being used to those that focus on peer support (Chapter 3), to the Dedicated Education Units that originated in Australia (Chapter 4) and the popular CLiP model that has seen prolific growth in the UK (Chapter 5). However, best practice continues to be led in Australia with the new clinical learning model of the Collaborative Clusters Education Model (CCEM) (Grealish et al., 2018). This model has been systematically and collaboratively evaluated during implementation using a reflexive methodology that responds to emerging concerns happening in real time clinical education.

Between 2016 and 2018, the School of Health and Education at Middlesex University, London has led on the two-year STEP (Strengthening Team-based Education in Practice) project to enhance learning in practice on behalf of and funded by Health Education England (HEE). This large collaborative initiative has been spearheaded by the practice-based learning team who have worked with professional programme teams, research centres, placement partners, three other local higher education institutes and student and service user groups.

In 2016, when the STEP project was in its infancy, the passion for practice learning was evident from the early debate and engagement that occurred between its members about the nature of practice learning. Each STEP member had an example of best practice and each could describe a placement that was unique to both the students and the staff that worked and learnt within it. This being the case, STEP debated whether it was possible to transfer clinical learning models seamlessly from one placement to the next or whether it would be better to support placements to achieve their own practice learning identity appropriate to their own students, service users and staff. As a consequence, STEP developed a strong socio-constructivist philosophy of promoting practice education collaboratively that used existing resources to enhance local and regional diversities.

One of the specific outcomes of the STEP project was the publication of this book which presents the five research steams of the project. These themes originated from the doctorate thesis of the external consultant for the STEP project (Morley, 2015) and previous unpublished HEE funded projects related to learning in practice that the team had worked upon. All five themes were identified for their importance to practice learning at this time.

The research-based approach to the book aims to give educators confidence for change in their own practice at a time when previous structures and guidance are being altered nationally.

Chapter 1 reviews literature focusing on the explicit value attached to both 'Comprehensive orientation and socialisation' in practice learning. The authors used focus groups to capture the thoughts and opinions of student nurses (n=41) from four higher education institutions. Students were asked four questions regarding preparation for and their experiences of the first two weeks of placement. The chapter analyses each of these questions in detail and explores the implications for teaching and learning within practice settings. The recommendations establish some principles of orientation, including the allocation of a named person, to ensure students are welcomed and established on placement as the first stage to their learning and socialisation.

Chapter 2, '"Helpful others": Recognising informal support networks for students in the clinical setting', examines the roles of people who help in the education of staff but who do not have a formal mentoring role (Eraut, 2007). In this chapter the teaching role of unregistered health care staff (health care assistants) is explored through focus groups with student nurses, mentors and health care assistants. The focus group questions were related to understanding of the health care assistant role in learning and teaching, the student experiences of working with health care assistants and how this occurs, the process and the value of feedback and learning together. Using thematic analysis to analyse the data, four main themes emerged: role relationships, accessibility, the experience of working with health care assistants and feedback. All groups recognised the value of health care assistants to the student experience of learning. Key findings suggest the need to develop a greater understanding of each other's roles and explicitly capture the value of the health care assistant regarding student learning, and how this transitions over time.

Chapter 3, 'Student peer support and learning', examines the literature on the value of peer learning and support in higher education. The first stage of this small-scale study was undertaken in August 2017 with Year 3 student nurses (n=19) and the second stage in May 2017 involving a group of midwifery (n= 7) and nursing students (n=5). The focus groups, with both nursing and midwifery student participants, explored their understanding and perceptions related to peer support and learning. Findings highlighted that junior peers benefitted from peer support, leading to reduced anxiety and increased learning opportunities in the practice setting. Recommendations highlighted the need for structured preparation and support across the student journey to ensure a peer approach is effective and valued throughout the curriculum. Guidance and examples of how this might be achieved are included.

Chapter 4 examines the need for robust 'Academic practice partnerships' required to deliver high quality and consistent education programmes for student nurses and midwives. A mixed methods approach was used to gather data from stakeholder participants. The findings from the data focused on six themes: preparation, roles, accessibility, networking, communication and expertise (PRANCE). Ongoing pressures in practice settings, and the need for protected staff time to undertake more effective learning and assessment, were highlighted in the research, as well as the need for clear communication, visibility, preparation and sharing learning opportunities. These competing demands have regularly been highlighted in the literature and this chapter will give guidance on navigating these. An analysis of current roles, the potential benefits and challenges of NMC new professional roles and recommendations to support new ways of working are explored.

Chapter 5 introduces 'Expansive learning' and the type of facilitation required to develop critical dialogue, reflexive expertise and leadership for learners. Expansive learning is led by the goal to discover what teaching and learning processes can assist all levels of clinical staff in supporting students to move effectively, and in a well-supported way, to the expertise or 'graduateness' required at registration and beyond. Data, to illicit views of what constitutes good coaching, was gathered in two phases: Phase 1 involved data collection from students via word cloud software, and Phase 2 involved three focus groups with mentors in a six-month study conducted in 2016–2017. Thematic analysis of the mentors' responses identified three themes key to supporting expansive learning in practice: 'Connecting', 'Establishing' and 'Expanding'. The empowerment of learners and building professional knowledge, skills and attributes were integral to the whole process. The resultant expansive learning coaching model is discussed at length in the chapter.

The book concludes with a summary of how the chapter findings and recommendations fit with the student journey through preparation for practice, practice itself and the application of learning back into the academic setting and students' longitudinal development. This includes relevant links to the NMC standards for nurses (NMC, 2018).

References

Baker, G. and Sheehy, K. (2017) The innovation of a fellowship role to promote mentor models in clinical practice for pre-registration nurses. *Health Education England*. Available at: https://www.hea cademy.ac.uk/system/files/hub/download/d2st10s6_gillian_baker.pdf (accessed 03/12/18).

Bazian. (2016) RCN mentorship project 2015. From today's support in practice to tomorrow's vision for excellence. *Royal College of Nursing*. Available at: https://www.rcn.org.uk/professiona l-development/publications/pub-005454 (accessed 10/08/18).

Council of Deans of Health. (2017a) CoDH response to NMC nurse education consultation. Available at: https://councilofdeans.org.uk/wp-content/uploads/2017/09/12092017-CoDH-Nurse-proficiencies-and-education-framework-consultation-response.pdf (accessed 06/12/18).

Council of Deans of Health. (2017b) Securing a sustainable future: Strategic plan 2018–2021. Available at: https://councilofdeans.org.uk/wp-content/uploads/2017/06/Strategic-plan-web-version.pdf (accessed 06/12/18).

Draper, J. and Kolyva, K. (2018) Carry on nursing! Education during turbulent times of change. RCN Education Forum National Conference and Exhibition 2018. Partners in Practice: Nurses Working Together Through Change.

Eraut, M. (2007) Learning from other people in the workplace, *Oxford Review of Education*, 33(4), pp. 403–422.

Grealish, L., Van de Mortel, T., Brown, C., Frommolt, V., Grafton, E., Havell, M., Needham, J., Shaw, J., Henderson, A. and Armit, L. (2018) Redesigning clinical education for nursing students and newly qualified nurses: A quality improvement study, *Nurse Education in Practice*, 33, pp. 84–89.

House of Commons (Health Select Committee). (2018) The nursing workforce. Available at: http s://publications.parliament.uk/pa/cm201719/cmselect/cmhealth/353/35304.htm#_idTextAn chor004 (accessed 12/03/2018).

Leigh, J. and Roberts, D. (2017) Implications for operationalising the new education standards for nursing, *British Journal of Nursing*, 26(21), pp. 1197–1199.

Leigh, J. and Roberts, D. (2018) Critical exploration of the new NMC standards of proficiency for registered nurses, *British Journal of Nursing*, 27(18), pp. 1068–1072.

Morley, D. A. (2015) A grounded theory study exploring first year student nurses' learning in practice. Doctor in Professional Practice thesis. Bournemouth, London: Bournemouth University.

Morley, D. A., Wilson, K. and McDermott, J. (2017) Changing the practice learning landscape, *Nurse Education in Practice*, 27, pp. 169–171.

Nursing and Midwifery Council (NMC). (2017) *Consultation on standards of proficiency for registered nurses*. Available at: https://www.nmc.org.uk/about-us/consultations/past-consultations/2017-consultations/ (accessed 03/15/19).

Nursing and Midwifery Council (NMC). (2018) NMC standards for nurses. Available at: https://www.nmc.org.uk/standards/standards-for-nurses/ (accessed 06/06/18).

Royal College of Nursing. (2017) Response to the NMC consultation on pre-registration standards and education. Available at: https://www.rcn.org.uk/professional-development/publica tions/pub-006447 (accessed 06/12/18).

Traverse. (2018) Evaluation of introduction of nursing associates: Phase 1 report for Health Education England. Available at: https://www.hee.nhs.uk/sites/default/files/documents/Phase% 201%20OPM%20Evaluation%20Report%20%28002%29.pdf (accessed 03/15/19).

UKCC. (1986) *Project 2000. A new preparation for practice*. London: UKCC.

Willis Commission. (2012) Quality with compassion: the future of nursing education. Report of the Willis Commission 2012: Executive summary. Available at: http://www.williscommission. org.uk (accessed 11/28/15).

Willis, G. (2015) Raising the bar. Shape of caring: A review of the future education and training of registered nurses and care assistants in England, London. Available at: https://www.hee.nhs.uk/ sites/default/files/documents/2348-Shape-of-caring-review-FINAL.pdf (accessed 03/15/19).

1 Comprehensive orientation and socialisation

*Lynn Quinlivan (l.t.1.quinlivan@herts.ac.uk),
Shoba Sookraj-Bahal, Julie Moody, Anne Levington and
Colin Taylor*

Introduction

Chapter 1 considers the importance of comprehensive orientation and socialisation in regard to the lived experiences of student nurses in four London hospitals in 2017.

Orientation is defined as the introduction to a new environment; it helps learners to adjust to these areas and eases them in their transition from university to their placement areas (Marcum and West, 2004; Charleston et al., 2007). In order for orientation to occur effectively there has to be an element of socialisation. Socialisation in nursing is about developing a professional identity (Zarshenas et al., 2014). It is where the learner becomes part of the team, adapts to their new environment and learns the necessary skills (Mackintosh, 2006). The two are therefore interdependent, and without orientation occurring then longer-term socialisation will be problematic.

The first two weeks in a clinical learning environment has, through custom and practice, been identified as the orientation phase. The remainder of the allocation is the time when learners more readily identified with active learning through the support of their practice supervisors and assessors. Consequently, this research study focuses on the learners' thoughts and perceptions of their first two weeks in a clinical learning environment.

Literature review

What is 'orientation and socialisation' in the context of practice learning?

Orientation and socialisation are far-reaching in their impact on how learners perceive that they are welcomed and supported in placement areas and provides an important foundation for their ongoing learning (Morley, 2015). Social learning theorists Lave and Wenger (1991) and Wenger (1998) discuss the importance of early socialisation into an occupational group so group members can become part of a functioning community of practice. Orientation and socialisation has a significant impact in helping students to decrease anxiety and improve their confidence and working relationship with staff (Cowen, Hubbard and Hancock, 2016) and decrease the risk of 'status dislocation' (Thomas, Jinks and Jack, 2015).

Watson et al. (2009) found that whilst the clinical area is deemed to be stressful, it plays a significant role in helping students to form a sense of belonging. Whilst it is acknowledged that orientation can be stressful for new learners commencing their nursing studies (Pearcy and Draper, 2008), it is also important to recognise that each placement experience can create its own anxieties for students.

Unfortunately, students' allocations do not always afford them the sense of permanence which would contribute to developing an identity. Clinical learning environments by their very nature are transient, with placement experiences ranging from a few days to several weeks. Brown, Stevens and Kermode (2012) felt that socialisation begins in the university setting, prior to students beginning placement, whilst Houghton (2014) argues that students don't really experience socialisation until they move into the clinical environment. Socialisation is, in fact, a long-term process which students experience throughout their academic and practice education as well as upon qualifying.

Despite its importance, research indicates inconsistencies in the way orientation is conducted for students (Castledine, 2002) and a lack of enquiry into seeking students' perspectives on their experiences. Lofmark and Wikblad (2001) and Levett-Jones, Lathlean and McMillan (2007) found that students do not always feel they fit into placement and can experience stress and worry due to the complexity of the experience. The Health Education England Recruitment and Retention project (HEE, 2018) emphasises the students' sense of vulnerability when the organisational culture does not embrace the individuality of a student. Dellasega et al. (2009) indicate that a lack of orientation is one of the contributory factors to attrition within nursing and that a positive orientation experience impacts on a student's decision to continue their studies and subsequently influences first destination post choice. Phillips, Esterman and Kenny (2015) also identify a correlation between a positive transition into a clinical placement and retention.

What are the importance and challenges of orientation and socialisation?

Building professional relationships from the outset is crucial to enabling a sense of belonging and psychological well-being to a developing learning experience. Staff who are welcoming and friendly contribute significantly to students feeling safe and confident (Spouse, 2000; Chesser-Smyth, 2005; Houghton et al., 2013; HEE, 2018). Levett-Jones et al. (2009b) identified that students attributed greater importance to being accepted, welcomed and part of the team than they did to the quality of patient care. Motivated learners who appeared to have a 'good' welcome to placement by friendly staff exhibited positive attitudes. Anxious students were deemed to have had a negative experience such as a poor welcome, lack of clear structure and staff who at the first point of contact were seen to be unfriendly (Levett-Jones et al., 2009b).

Jackson et al. (2011) found that students in some placement areas felt unwelcome, ignored and invisible as staff did not make the time to welcome or engage them in learning activities. This resulted in a feeling of dissatisfaction at the end of their nurse education, which students felt was due to poor socialisation and acceptance into their allocated placement areas. Stress related behaviours were also apparent. If students found that they were not expected on placement, this evoked a sense of loss and bewilderment which was not easily remedied (Allan, Smith and Lorentzon, 2008). The psychological effect upon the learner is well documented with feelings of isolation and anxiety (Papp, Markkanen and von Bondsroff, 2003).

Davey (2002) found permanent staff felt that having a student to support created more work for the nursing team particularly when they were short staffed. This is echoed by Lopez et al. (2018) who outlines that students expressed the opinion that staff were at times unsupportive and hesitant to teach learners new and increasingly complicated skills. This was in part due to registered nurses having their own personal anxieties about their capabilities to teach, alongside individual students' ability to perform safely and competently under supervision. Yet, despite this, students felt that staff contributed significantly to what they learnt in clinical practice and their socialisation into the placement environment (Baldwin et al., 2014).

When a sense of belonging is not developed, students will (out of a sense of self-preservation and the need to be accepted) provide care that may be acceptable by staff in the placement although not identified as good practice (Walker et al., 2011). Furthermore, the learner will devote time and energy to trying to become part of the team and to 'fit in' rather than focus on their individual learning needs (Lofmark and Wikblad, 2001).

The nuances of how staff support students are therefore important as they can either have a positive or negative effect on the learner at an individual or collective level, which subsequently impinges on the student's ability to develop clinical competence, confidence and critical thinking.

What are the elements of good orientation and socialisation?

For students to be socialised appropriately to a clinical learning environment area, several key elements need to be routinely considered, namely: a structured and meaningful orientation with a positive attitude and ward culture which embraces learners (Pearcy and Elliot, 2004). Staff attitude is highly significant, and research indicates inconsistency with students; some felt useless and undervalued whilst others relished being a respected part of the team (Bradbury-Jones, Sambrook and Irvine, 2011; Walker et al., 2014). Wenger (1998), Gherardi, Nicolini and Odella (1998), Grealish and Ranse (2009) and Chesser-Smyth (2005) established that learners being able to independently perform certain tasks and skills prepared them better for practice, improving their confidence and helping them to feel useful in practice.

Role models who exhibit positive attributes both in terms of professional behaviours and clinical abilities are important (Woodward, 2003) and can assist students to deal with difficulties or challenges they may experience (Filstad, 2004). Walker et al. (2014) attributes positive role modelling to students feeling a sense of belonging. Being included as part of the team builds a student's sense of self-worth, feelings of acceptance and an increase in their confidence and willingness to take an enquiry-based approach to their own learning. Unregistered health care workers are quite significant in helping students to orientate and settle in but even this can end in dissatisfaction if they felt threatened by the learners (Castledine, 2002).

Time is another factor that can affect the practice staff's ability to orientate learners and student peer support on the first day of placement can reduce anxiety and allow learners to learn from their peers they meet on placement (Reeve et al., 2013). Research by Lopez et al. (2018) found that learners felt speaking to their peers reduced individual stress and consequently made the learner feel emotionally supported. Morley (2015) recommends that students start a new placement at a time when workload is reduced and staff have more time to spend orientating the student with less clinical distractions.

In conclusion, a structured orientation leads to greater student satisfaction and an ability to grasp new learning opportunities (Thomas et al., 2015; Levett-Jones et al., 2009b; Chesser-Smyth, 2005), but the authors found limited research on how this could be achieved through the student perspective.

Methodology

In order to understand the lived experiences of learners, a research study was undertaken which sought to capture the thoughts and opinions of student nurses drawn from four higher educational institutions (HEI) across five practice organisations in London. The aim of the study was to elicit the thoughts and opinions of student nurses in clinical practice with regards to their experiences of orientation and socialisation, with reference to the first two weeks in a new placement.

Ethical approval was granted from the University's Ethics Committee. Forty-one student participants were recruited to the focus groups via an electronic invitation. Students who responded to the invitation were provided with information about informed consent and their ongoing confidentiality and anonymity from the research (NMC, 2015). The two focus group events occurred in January and February 2017.

As established in the literature review, comprehensive orientation has the potential to significantly impact on a learner regardless of the stage in their education. Consequently, all learners studying one of the four fields of nursing, namely adult, child, mental health and learning disability, were invited to take part in one of the two focus group events. The first event comprised of ten students from different fields of nursing located at two tables and students were requested not to sit at a table where there was an academic representative from their own HEI in order to prevent unconscious bias in the case of both students and facilitators. The second event was held in a lecture theatre with a mixed group of 31 students.

The focus group participants were asked four key questions:

1 Prior to placement what best prepared you for practice?
2 During the first two weeks of placement what was most helpful for your orientation?
3 Who were most helpful during your first two weeks in your clinical placement?
4 What could have been better during the first two weeks?

At the first event, student participants discussed the questions written on the flip charts and were encouraged to add to the data by means of Post-it Notes. Each group was supported by a member of the research team who facilitated the discussion whilst another member of the team took field notes, to ensure that the conversation between students was effectively captured. At the second event, flip charts with the key questions were attached to the walls of the lecture theatre, and learners were able to move freely between the charts adding their thoughts and opinions onto Post-it Notes. This activity was then followed by an oral discussion facilitated by a member of the research team, and additional oral comments were captured in the form of field notes by a member of the research team.

Qualitative data was analysed by the research team according to the responses to each question.

Results

To ensure accuracy and reliability of the thematic process, the authors independently coded the data generated under the lead questions. Reoccurring themes, along with supportive quotations, are presented in the following pages.

Question 1:
Prior to placements, what best prepared you for your practice?

The students' narrative covered three broad areas, namely accuracy, timeliness of information and first impressions.

The four HEIs all used differing placement allocation systems to disseminate information to both students and clinical staff, and it became apparent that there was no standardisation in regards to either the length of time that students knew about their placement in advance or "contact information which was current and timely" (focus group 1).

Strategies that involved an increased sense of control were welcomed, from receiving ward information packs to listening to talks by more senior students on what to expect and "being able to email the placements to introduce myself and get more information about the area" (focus group 1). Other students appreciated the "opportunity to develop competency with skills in advance of placement feeling more confident prior to allocation" (focus group 2). The underlying theme of off duty not being readily available was recognised as a key stressor.

Students in focus group 2 did highlight the appreciation and value of receiving and having access to online induction information, though it was raised as an actual experience by a minority number of the group. Interestingly, the remaining students within the group felt this was a good idea and would have liked to have had access to online resources had this option made available to them.

The discussion moved on from timeliness of information to first impressions. What was apparent from the students' narrative was that the underlying principle of feeling welcomed and acknowledged is as relevant for students new to an area as it is for patients, clients and service users. For students, the first point of contact did not need to be their nominated practice supervisor or practice assessor. The most effective support often came from unregistered health care staff. The theme "Welcoming environment and a key person to latch onto" (focus group 2) along with "Having HCAs [health care assistants] or students to orientate and make you feel comfortable" (focus group 1) clearly indicate that for orientation to be effective a nominated individual is crucial.

Question 2:
During the first two weeks of placement, what was most helpful for your orientation?

The role of the mentor in supporting learning and assessment in practice (NMC, 2008) was frequently highlighted by the students. Although the term 'mentor' has been used throughout this research conducted in 2017, the terminology will change to that of 'practice supervisor' and 'practice assessor' in line with the NMC (2018) Standards for Student Supervision and Assessment from 2019 onwards. The overarching principle of a knowledgeable individual being present and supporting learners will remain pivotal to a quality learning experience, for example, "Making sure you are allocated a mentor who is actually there, so you can 'latch' on to somebody" (focus group 1).

Undoubtedly, structure was fundamental to a successful orientation. "In my current placement, the staff were aware that a student was coming and I felt a lot more welcomed and accepted. I only had two placements that did this" (focus group 1).

Yet again the role of health care support workers was viewed as being important to the learner's socialisation. "Having HCAs or other students already there to orientate and make you feel comfortable" (focus group 2).

Data found that students wanted the initial interview in a timely manner with some negotiation for the future management of their placement. "Having a full day of orientation, meeting most of the mentors and doing the initial interview within the first week – being allowed to be involved in planning my rota" (focus group 2).

Question 3:
Who were most helpful during your first two weeks in your clinical placement?

Students began to attribute key characteristics of titles and roles to those who were deemed to be most help. The mentor who was newly registered or who had considerable experience was able to provide a higher level of support and guidance: "Two newly registered nurses on the ward who understood exactly how I felt and what I would and wouldn't already have learned" (focus group 2). Students also identified that they themselves could provide self-help: "myself". Receiving timely information again was seen as being valuable in enabling and empowering the student to actively prepare for the clinical learning environment and thereby have an understanding of naturally occurring learning opportunities.

Question 4:
What factors would have enhanced your first two weeks in practice?

Themes that emerged related to expectations of students and staff supporting learners in clinical learning environments.

From the students' perspective, a structured orientation enabled them to identify skills which they had yet to acquire. Without a structured orientation, and clear identification of a named individual to complete the summative assessments, learners felt that they were expected to undertake skills outside their sphere of knowledge and practice or were deprived of learning opportunities, "being shown how to do something . . . don't assume what we can/can't do" (focus group 1). Making time and support were important, "giving specific learning objective and allow student to have time to do and demonstrate" (focus group 2), particularly when the learning environment was found to be either busy or functioning at less than an optimum level in respect to the staff-patient ratio.

One striking theme that emerged was the style and manner of nurse leadership and the impact that this had upon the clinical learning environment both in terms of patient care and a team's ability to manage workload. A direct association was made between positive role models and student satisfaction with their learning:

"Staff (mainly sisters) working together with students rather than putting their frustration on them and sticking to positive attitudes – better leadership" (focus group 1).

"Mentors to help with arranging opportunities more – students often dismissed" (focus group 2).

Analysis

From both the literature review, and results from the focus groups, it is evident that themes such as sense of belonging, learner anxiety and time to learn continue to resonate

(Cowen et al., 2016; Watson et al., 2009; Allan et al., 2008). The impact of positive role models, along with a structured orientation to the clinical learning environment, has been identified by Thomas et al. (2015), and the data analysis concurs with this study's findings. Support from others, such as peers or registered nurses not necessarily identified as a named mentor, has been shown to be effective (Levett-Jones and Lathlean, 2009a), and this chapter has identified also the role of the unregistered health care assistant as relevant to contribute to students' sense of belonging or as a teaching and learning resource.

Students focused on the characteristics of the person or persons who provided a positive orientation, such as "welcoming, latch onto and key individual" (focus group 2) rather than their status in the clinical setting. Vinales (2015) highlighted the role of the mentor and the pivotal impact that this role has on the student's journey. At the time that the research was conducted the NMC (2008) standards were in place. One of the standards was that learners should be supervised by their named mentor directly or indirectly for 40 per cent of their time within the clinical learning environment. It is concerning that students felt the need to use such emotive language as "find someone to latch onto" (focus group 2). Although not explicitly linked to the desire to 'fit in' (Melia, 1987; Morley, 2015) this highlights the continued risk of learners adapting taught standards of care to short cuts or behaviour learnt by rote that may have become insidious in practice (Morley, 2015).

The value of orientation packs (Reynolds and Kaur, 2016), explanation by more senior students and the ability to contact placement, or to practice clinical skills prior to placement, built confidence going into the clinical environment. This proved an essential precursor to students' experience.

Although the findings cannot necessarily be generalised to all student nurses, one common theme of note is the conflict that students expressed with regards to balancing learning opportunities, clinical demands and time to learn, showing that Allan et al's (2008) findings still resonate with learners a decade on. What students did not vocalise is the emotional toll that this decision-making process had upon them (Grealish and Ranse, 2009) nor whether this impacted upon their choice of first destination post.

Conclusion

The findings from this research study indicate that central to a meaningful orientation and a student's ability to become socialised into a clinical learning environment is undoubtedly the manner in which the student is welcomed and supported during their orientation. Key to providing students with a valuable and meaningful learning experience is to acknowledge their lived experiences and address, through structured orientation, how they become socialised into the clinical learning environment and ultimately the future workforce. This occurs both before the placement experience and a significant period of time afterwards and is individual to their own personal experience.

Clarity of learning opportunities via the mechanisms of a structured orientation enables the learner to develop not only a sense of identity, and thus belonging, but also the confidence to take an inquiry-based approach to their own learning. Students identify themselves as a significant resource to orientation, but this should be complementary to planned structures made both before and during placement. A greater use of online information to orientate the student to the placement and their staff could, for example, be further mobilised to ensure a consistent and quality led approach.

The influence and support of a named member of staff is key, and the provision by unregistered health care support workers (HCAs) requires formal acknowledgement rather than the 'ad hoc' process that currently exists. The role of the HCAs in the process of students' learning is further discussed in Chapter 2, '"Helpful others" – recognising informal support networks for students in the clinical setting'. Likewise, Chapter 3 identifies the potential of peer students, at different points in their educational journey, for mutual learning to occur during the placement induction period.

The research could be further enhanced by conducting focus groups with students at the two-week point going into placement, as this proved too difficult to achieve on this occasion. The authors also recognise the limitations of the study which was undertaken with a group of learners who were commissioned and in receipt of a bursary. Since the study was completed student nurses and midwives are now required to pay fees and take out student loans. What would be interesting to establish is the thoughts and opinions of learners who are affected by this fundamental shift in UK government policy. The opinions of learners entering nursing studies in the UK by other routes, such as nursing degree apprenticeships, have not yet been captured by research studies.

Recommendations

1. Establish principles of good orientation in the practice setting

Information to assist contact between academic and clinical staff who support student learning is identified in Chapter 4. It is recommended that each practice setting, in conjunction with their academic colleagues, provide key contact information, the profile of placement and the structure of clinical teams, appropriate to a student's individual and programme orientation. A consistency in approach across the organisation would begin to mitigate against the present diversity of student experience.

2. Identify a key person who takes responsibility for a student's individual orientation

Analysis of findings from the focus groups indicates that students' ability to integrate into the clinical learning environment stems from orientation being conducted by a named person. That key person does not, from the students' point of view, need to be a registered health professional. The role of unregistered staff or more advanced peers could be actively considered across the organisation and the demarcation of skills from both registered and unregistered staff to complement a more holistic and social learning approach to student induction.

3. Careful selection of the practice supervisor

The value of recently registered nurses being nominated as a supervisor again stems from the findings. Students vocalised that newly registered nurses had a greater understanding of their lived experiences and thus were able to identify learning opportunities which were both relevant and timely. It is recommended that clinical leads, with increased management responsibilities, support registered staff with greater availability and possible connection with students.

4. Evaluate whether the clinical learning environment is welcoming to learners

As this chapter has explored, key to students' ability to embrace learning opportunities is a sense of belonging and socialisation into the learning environment team. It is recommended that students are encouraged to exercise their voice to evaluate their orientation experience at their official learning review points on placement.

Case study for comprehensive orientation and socialisation

Claire is a first-year student who is about to start her first placement area in four weeks. The Higher Education Institute (HEI) has sent all the names of the students to the placements four weeks in advance. Claire has never been to this practice organisation and is anxious about what to expect when she commences placement.

What is the learning aim?

To increase meaningful and structured orientation to placement that allows a positive and safe start to practice learning.

What learning will be achieved?

At the end of week two Claire will have a defined orientation to practice and will be able to identify individuals who are providing supporting structures to assist with her ongoing socialisation.

How can learning be supported?

1 Preparation for transition into practice that welcomes Claire before she starts

Learners who are made to feel welcome when they arrive on practice placement experience a reduction of stress and anxiety (Levett-Jones et al., 2009b). Best practice is that organisations identify and continuously develop expertise of a named coordinator of learners for each placement. One of the roles of the coordinator is to send Claire a welcome letter, which includes her supervisor's name, an initial rota for discussion, start and finish times as well as whom to ask for on her first day. The placement's orientation pack sets the scene for the client groups that Claire will deliver care to. This will give Claire clarity and structure, and thus a sense of belonging within the practice organisation, and allow independent preparation for some of the conditions that she may meet.

2 Establishment of a team of induction staff to support the learners on placement

Cowen et al. (2016) found that learners judged how friendly staff members were by the welcome that they received when they started their placement. The named person on Claire's first day will have the responsibility to introduce Claire to all team members and explain their roles and responsibilities as part of a structured orientation. This will enable Claire to gain a wider understanding of context and nature of care provided, naturally occurring learning opportunities and clarity in respect to her role and responsibilities as a first-year learner. This is an opportunity for the supervisor to establish Claire's prior learning and therefore identify learning opportunities with appropriate prepared professionals.

3 Creation of a positive learning culture within each practice placement

Evidence suggests one of the most important aspects of a positive placement is whether or not, the learner feels that they belong in the setting (Baldwin et al., 2014; Vinales, 2015). Best practice is that a named co-coordinator of learners would identify a practice assessor who demonstrates positive engagement with a novice learner such as Claire. This demonstrates that the coordinator has a rationale for allocating the appropriate team members to the assessor, thereby ensuring that Claire experiences aspects of well-being explicitly linked to the term socialisation such as 'sense of belonging'.

References

Allan, H.T., Smith, P.A. and Lorentzon, M. (2008) Leadership for learning: A literature study of leadership for learning in clinical practice, *Journal of Nursing Management*, 16(50), pp. 545–555.

Baldwin, A., Mills, J., Birks, M. and Budden, L. (2014) Role modelling in undergraduate nursing education: An integrative literature review, *Nurse Education Today*, 34(6), pp. e18–e26.

Bradbury-Jones, C. Sambrook, S. and Irvine, F. (2011) Empowerment and being valued: A phenomenological study of nursing students' experiences of clinical practice, *Nurse Education Today*, 31(4), pp. 368–372.

Brown, J., Stevens, J. and Kermode, S. (2012) Measuring student nurse professional socialisation: The development and implementation of a new instrument, *Nurse Education Today*, 33 (6), pp. 565–573.

Castledine, G. (2002) Student must be treated better in clinical areas, *British Journal of Nursing*, 11 (18), pp. 1222–1222.

Charleston, R., Hayman-White, K., Ryan, R. and Hapell, B. (2007) Understanding the importance of effective orientation: What does this mean in psychiatric graduate nurse programs? *Australian Journal of Advanced Nursing*, 25(1), pp. 24–30.

Chesser-Smyth, P.A. (2005) The lived experience of general student nurses on their first clinical placement: A phenomenological study, *Nurse Education in Practice*, 5(5), pp. 320–327.

Cowen, J. K., Hubbard, L.J. and Hancock, D.C. (2016) Concerns of nursing students beginning clinical courses: A descriptive study, *Nurse Education Today*, 43, pp. 64–68.

Davey, L. (2002) Nurses eating nurses: The caring profession which fails to nurture its own, *Contemporary Nurse*, 13(2–3), pp. 192–197.

Dellasega, C., Gabbay, R., Durdock, K. and Martinez-King, N. (2009) An exploratory study of the orientation needs of experienced nurses, *Journal of Continuing Education in Nursing*, 40(7), pp. 311–316.

Filstad, C. (2004) How newcomers use role models in organisational socialisation, *Journal of Workplace Learning*, 16(7), pp. 396–409.

Gherardi, S., Nicolini, D. and Odella, F. (1998) Toward a social understanding of how people learn in organizations: The notion of situated curriculum, *Management Learning*, 29(3), pp. 273–297.

Grealish, L. and Ranse, K. (2009) An exploratory study of first year nursing students' learning in the clinical workplace, *Contemporary Nurse*, 33(1), pp. 80–92.

Health Education England (HEE). (2018) RePAIR: Reducing Pre-Registration Attrition and Improving Retention Report. Available at: https://www.hee.nhs.uk/our-work/reducing-pre-registration-attrition-improving-retention (accessed 02/11/18).

Houghton, C.E. (2014) 'Newcomer adaptation': A lens through which to understand how nursing students fit in with the real world of practice, *Journal of Clinical Nursing*, 23(15–16), pp. 2367–2375.

Houghton, C., Casey, D., Shaw, D. and Murphy, K. (2013) Students' experiences of implementing clinical skills in the real world of practice, *Journal of Clinical Nursing*, 22(13–14), pp. 1961–1969.

Jackson, D., Hutchinson, M., Everett, B., Mannix, J., Peters, K., Weaver, R. and Salamonson, Y. (2011) Struggling for legitimacy: Nursing students' stories of organisational aggression, resilience and resistance, *Nursing Inquiry*, 18(2), pp. 102–110.

Lave, J. and Wenger, E. (1991) *Situated learning: Legitimate Peripheral Participation*. Cambridge, UK: Cambridge University Press.

Levett-Jones, T., Lathlean, J. and McMillan, M. (2007) The duration of clinical placements: a key influence on nursing students' experience of belongingness, *Australian Journal of Advanced Nursing*, 26(2), pp. 8–16.

Levett-Jones, T. and Lathlean, J. (2009a) 'Don't rock the boat': Nursing students' experiences of conformity and compliance, *Nurse Education Today*, 29(3), pp. 342–349.

Levett-Jones, T., Lathlean, J., Higgins, I. and McMillan, M. (2009b) Staff-student relationship and their impact on nursing students' belongingness and learning, *Journal of Advanced Nursing*, 65(2), pp. 316–324.

Lofmark, A. and Wikblad, K. (2001) Facilitating and obstructing factors for development of learning in clinical practice: a student perspective, *Journal of Advanced Nursing*, 34(1), pp. 43–50.

Lopez, V., Yobas, P., Leng Chow, Y. and Shorey, S. (2018) Does building resilience in undergraduate nursing students happen through clinical placements? A qualitative study, *Nurse Education Today*, 67, pp. 1–5.

Mackintosh, C. (2006) Caring: the socialisation of pre-registration student nurses: A longitudinal qualitative descriptive study, *International Journal of Nursing Studies*, 43(8), pp. 953–962.

Marcum, E. and West, R. (2004) Structured orientation for new graduates: A retention strategy, *Journal for Nurses in Staff Development*, 20(3), pp. 118–124.

Melia, K. (1987) *Learning and working: The occupational socialisation of nurses*. London: Tavistock.

Morley, D.A. (2015) A grounded theory study exploring first year student nurses' learning in practice. Doctor in Professional Practice thesis. Bournemouth, UK: Bournemouth University.

Nursing and Midwifery Council (NMC). (2008) *Standards to support learning and assessment in practice*. London: Nursing and Midwifery Council.

Nursing and Midwifery Council (NMC). (2015) *Professional standards of practice and behaviour for nurses, midwives and nursing associates*. London: Nursing and Midwifery Council. Available at: https://www.nmc.org.uk/globalassets/sitedocuments/nmc-publications/nmc-code.pdf (accessed 10/21/18).

Nursing and Midwifery Council (NMC). (2018) *Standards for student supervision and assessment*. London: Nursing and Midwifery Council. Available at: https://www.nmc.org.uk/globalassets/sitedocuments/na-consultation/standards-for-student-supervision-and-assessment.pdf (accessed 10/21/18).

Papp, M., Markkanen, M., and von Bondsdroff, M. (2003) Clinical environment as a learning environment: student nurses' perception concerning clinical learning environment, *Nurse Education Today*, 23(4), pp. 262–267.

Pearcy, P. and Elliot, B. (2004) Student impressions of clinical nursing, *Nurse Education Today*, 24(5), pp. 382–387.

Pearcy, P. and Draper, P. (2008) Exploring clinical nursing experiences: Listening to student nurses, *Nurse Education Today*, 28(5), pp. 595–601.

Phillips, C., Esterman, A. and Kenny, A. (2015) The theory of organisational socialisation and its potential for improving transition experiences for new graduate nurses, *Nurse Education Today*, 35(1), pp. 118–124.

Reeve, K.L., Shumaker, C.J., Yearwood, E.L., Crowell, N.A. and Riley, J.B. (2013) Perceived stress and social support in undergraduate nursing students' educational experiences, *Nurse Education Today*, 33(4), pp. 419–424.

Reynolds, S. and Kaur, R. (2016) Supporting nurses with an online induction, *Nursing Times*, 112 (45/46), pp. 13–15.

Spouse, J. (2000) Bridging theory and practice in the supervisory relationship: A sociocultural perspective, *Journal of Advanced Nursing*, 33(4), pp. 512–522.

Thomas, J., Jinks, A. and Jack, B. (2015) Finessing incivility: The professional socialisation experiences of a student nurses' first clinical placement, a grounded theory, *Nurse Education Today*, 35(12), pp. e4–e9.

Vinales, J.J. (2015) The mentor as a role model and the importance of belongingness, *British Journal of Nursing*, 24(10), pp. 532–535.

Walker, R., Henderson, A., Cooke, M. and Creedy, D. (2011) Impact of a learning circle intervention across academic and service contexts on developing a learning culture, *Nurse Education Today*, 31(4), pp. 378–382.

Walker, S., Dwyer, T., Broadbent, M., Moxham, L. and Sander, S. (2014) Constructing a nursing identity within the clinical environment: The student nurse experience, *Contemporary Nurse*, 49 (1), pp. 103–112.

Watson, R., Gardinier, E., Houghton, R., Gibson, H., Stimson, A., Wrate, R. and Deary, I. (2009) A longitudinal study of stress and psychological distress in nurses and nursing students, *Journal of Clinical Nursing*, 18(2), pp. 270–278.

Wenger, E. (1998) *Communities of practice: Learning, meaning and identity*. New York: Cambridge University Press.

Woodward, W. (2003) Preparing a new workforce, *Nursing Administration Quarterly*, 27(3), pp. 215–222.

Zarshenas, L., Sharif, F., Molazem, Z., Khayyer, M., Zare, N. and Ebadi, A. (2014) Professional socialisation in nursing: A qualitative content analysis, *Iranian Journal of Nursing and Midwifery Research*, 19(4), pp. 432–443.

2 'Helpful others': Recognising support networks for students in the clinical setting

Pam Hodge (p.hodge@mdx.ac.uk), Alison Dexter and Helen O'Toole

Introduction

Care in the 21st century is delivered by a diverse team, comprising unregistered and registered staff. This can include student nurses and midwives, providing opportunities to work and learn together with permanent staff. Chapter 2 explores how this social learning is achieved from the perspective of different learners in practice.

Eraut (2007) coined the term 'Helpful Others' to encompass the valuable contributions to education made by the wider team, not officially acknowledged for their input. Nursing students in practice are regularly supported by health care assistants (Hasson, 2013). The extent to which this happens and how this is monitored varies between placement areas. Therefore, good and bad practice goes 'under the radar' resulting in potential quality variance.

Professional bodies in the UK require student learning in practice to be formally assessed by an individual on the same part of the register (NMC, 2018a); however, there is limited documented knowledge of other professionals, outside of nursing, where learners in practice are regularly supported by unregistered staff. This research acknowledges the importance of exploring the relationship between learners in practice and health care assistants, including trainee nursing associates whose role is intended to address a skills gap between health care assistants and registered nurses. The nursing associate role, introduced in England in 2017, aims to be a 'bridging one between healthcare support workers and graduate registered nurses, and aims to support the career progression of care assistants, increase the supply of nurses and enable nurses to undertake more advanced roles' (Traverse, 2018, p. 1). For this research we have adopted the term 'health care assistant' (HCA) to refer to all care assistants in the team including healthcare assistants, advanced practitioners, support workers, and trainee nursing associates.

Willis (2015), Bazian (2016) and Cavendish (2013) comment that most of the direct patient care is provided by HCAs with 315,000 in post in the UK in September 2017 (NHS Digital, 2018). The role of the HCA is varied and their responsibilities within each clinical area can differ vastly within the same service provider (Padfield and Knowles, 2014).

To understand if the HCA cohort can be considered as 'Helpful Others', a review of the literature informed the shaping of the focus group questions to explore the experiences of students, mentors, and HCAs in practice.

Literature review

What is the role of the HCA in practice education?

The supernumerary role of the student in practice, coupled with the increasing roles and responsibilities of the registered nurse, has led to the expansion of the role of the healthcare support workers, who now undertake certain work that would previously have been carried out by registered staff. Willis (2015) and Sarre et al. (2018) reported that health care assistants currently provide approximately 60 per cent of hands-on care. This is supported by the findings of Unison (2010) where they acknowledge that HCAs are often responsible for the fundamentals of patient care. In doing so they often work alone with little or no access to supervision, undertaking tasks that are traditionally associated with registered nurse work including administration of medication. Despite the increasing responsibilities of the HCA, Willis (2015, p. 36), found 'many care assistants feel undervalued and overlooked.'

There is growing acknowledgement of the extensive number of clinical practice skills that student nurses can learn from HCAs (Padfield and Knowles, 2014). The role of the HCA in helping to support learners in clinical placement has been recognised in the literature, (Thornley, 2000; O'Driscoll, Allan, and Smith, 2010). Hasson, McKenna, and Keeney (2012) and Hasson (2013) shows the diversity of the roles of the unregistered workforce, recognising their differing skills and their input into pre-registration practice education.

Registered nurses acknowledge that their increased clinical workload affects the support and learning experience they provide to students (Gray and Smith, 2000; Myall, Levett-Jones, and Lathlean, 2008). This concurs with Morley's (2018) findings that student nurses recognise the possibility of their learning being compromised due to the competing demands on the mentors in practice.

It seems that HCAs have stepped into this divide, but, despite training and increased responsibilities undertaken by the HCA, the registered nurse remains accountable for the students' clinical education (NMC, 2018a) to ensure safe and effective service user care. The juxtaposition of HCA to contribute to student nurse education, without training for their own roles, was recognised in the 2014 Francis Report and led to the recommendations of the 2015 Cavendish Report that training and regulation were needed for the HCA workforce.

Is there any value to the HCA and learners in practice working together?

Hasson et al. (2012, p. 229) found that 'nurse training did not sufficiently prepare students for the realities of clinical practice' with learners discussing the fears and barriers they encountered when faced with delegating tasks. This included not being given the opportunity to work independently in a supervisory situation (Bisholt et al., 2014).

Opportunities to practice these skills can occur through working with HCAs in practice. Thus, the relationship between students and HCAs may change over time; initially students learn practical skills from the HCA, and as their training progresses, the learners may delegate these same skills to the HCAs, thus gaining experience and development of a different set of skills. Padfield and Knowles (2014) highlight areas where nursing students in practice valued and supported the role of the unregistered practitioner in their learning, referring to it as 'unregistered mentorship'. They recommended the use of specified frameworks to ensure the quality of mentorship, assessment of learner experiences, and that unregistered practitioners, undertaking this enhanced role, should be recognised with accreditation.

Annear, Lea, and Robinson (2014) found that students, and the HCAs teaching them, benefited from a specific support framework for assessing personal care following the development of a 'Carer Assessment and Reporting Guide'. HCAs reported feeling valued and students' appreciation of personal care skills were enhanced.

What are the challenges to HCAs helping students with their learning in practice?

Willis (2015) found that the interaction between the learners and the HCAs did not reflect the whole range of possible learning opportunities. Hasson et al. (2012) and Hasson (2013) highlight the involvement of the HCA as unstructured, usually on an 'ad hoc' basis and undertaken both with and without approval of registered nurses when mentors are unavailable. Clarke's (2015) study found learners, undertaking clinical placements in the independent sector, reported a 'silo' model of working where they learnt specific tasks from the HCAs and specific tasks from the registered nurses. Within this model of working, the learners may not always have opportunity to work with the HCAs. If there were enough HCAs on duty the HCA would decline the 'help' from the learners, resulting in the learner being unable to observe the task being performed. This finding was further explored by Johnson et al. (2015) and Morley (2018) who found that the working relationship between registered nurses and healthcare assistants differed, some working successfully together whilst others work 'in parallel'. They recommended that newly registered nurses required more assistance in developing working relationships with HCAs.

Gillespie and Rivers (2017) also recognise the contribution of HCAs to the development of students in practice. They believe that the reluctance to formalise a collaborative team approach complicates nursing education, resulting in the learner finding it more challenging to develop their own professional identity. This challenge is accentuated by a lack of defined role for unregistered staff. Bungay, Jackson, and Lord (2016) found that the role of the assistant practitioner was referred to by many different job titles, and a greater level of clarity was needed by registered practitioners. Potential role drift (Padfield and Knowles, 2014) contributed to confusion of roles and accountability. The experience of HCAs therefore varies significantly, and it is vital that registered nurses can recognise the diversity within the HCA workforce (Burrow, Gilmour, and Cook, 2017) and support learners to navigate this complex practice picture.

Students have often gained experience of working as an HCA prior to embarking on their university education. The positive influence of past experience on the socialisation process is highlighted by Morley (2018) although challenges exist whereby students, with HCA experience, may find that their ability to undertake the work may be detrimental to their contrasting role as a learner.

Methodology

To gain an understanding of the relationship between students and HCAs and how it changes over time (Hasson et al., 2012), it was decided to use a qualitative methodology. Ethical approval was granted from the University's Ethics Committee. There was an acknowledgement of the power differentials and risk of coercion for those taking part in the research.

The literature search informed the development of six semi-structured questions:

1   What do you perceive as the role of helpful others, including HCA whilst you are on your placement? What is their role is supporting student nurses?
2   Describe the structure of your experience of working with HCAs. Is this decided by your mentor, the HCA, yourself, or in a different way?
3   How do you feel about working with HCAs? How does this differ from working with your mentor?
4   What feedback do you receive working with a HCA, and when? Is this feedback directed to yourself? What form does this take – verbal/documented? How do they assess it? Against what?
5   How would you describe the value of working with HCAs? Please give one aspect of working with HCAs that is most relevant to your education.
6   We would like to create a useful toolkit with ideas and resources that could support learners and HCAs. What would you like to suggest would be useful to include in this toolkit to maximise the benefits of working with HCAs?

Focus groups were undertaken by the authors between January–June 2017 to obtain the primary data set and were conducted by researchers as either a small or large group discussion of the questions. The discussions were captured in the majority by audio recordings unless specified.

The focus groups consisted of the following:

1   Students. The student focus groups were purposively sampled by year of study. The whole population of students in practice at the time of the focus groups were invited to attend and represented all fields of nursing and midwifery and related their experiences to inpatient, outpatient, and community settings. These three focus groups all took place in the final week of their placements between January and May 2017. This included a group at the end of their first clinical placement (n=6) to capture very early in education perceptions, and two groups from Year 2 (n=9) and Year 3 (n=5).
2   Mentors (n=75) were purposefully sampled at three practice learning conferences and three focus groups conducted as a result.
3   Health care assistants.

    HCA focus group one: HCAs (n=4) had completed their care certificate and expressed an interest in supporting students.
    HCA focus group two: HCAs (n=25) attended a practice led event about supporting students and volunteered for the study. HCAs were asked for their responses on flipcharts whilst taking an author took field notes.
    HCA focus group three: HCAs (n=50) attended a practice induction about supporting students and volunteered for the study. HCAs were asked for their responses on flipcharts whilst taking an author took field notes.

4   Trainee nursing associates (TNAs) (n=10) were recruited at two TNA forums. One of the authors asked TNAs to complete a questionnaire based on the focus group questions.

The existing literature (Zaitseva, Milsom, and Stewart, 2013) demonstrated there is a change in the relationship between HCA and learners at some point in their education.

It was not clear when this transition occurs and by undertaking the focus groups at strategic times, it was hoped this change could be identified.

All the data was analysed thematically by the authors, and four themes emerged (Table 2.1).

Results and analysis

1. Role relationships

Perceptions of the HCA roles vary within practice areas (Bosley and Dale, 2008), and the students' level of education. Due to the large variance in the role of HCA, role confusion can occur. The HCAs also reported the need for clarity of learners' roles and learning needs at each stage of educational programmes.

In the student focus groups, when asked their understanding of the HCA role, responses were vague: "They help nurses to do their job" (Year 1, student nurse). The HCAs also reported that students were not informed of the HCA roles beyond personal care and unaware of the complex clinical tasks increasingly being undertaken by the HCA.

Whilst everyone was busy, "the HCAs are always there for you" (Year 1, student nurse). The HCAs reported that the students regularly worked with them and some specifically involved students in activities which were beyond routine and offered valuable learning opportunities such as in a clinical emergency. As students progressed through the course the relationship with the HCAs altered and became more dichotomous; there was a greater understanding of the role and acknowledgement of the importance of the HCAs to their learning, "Without the HCAs it would not be possible to do a lot of things – they do the hard work – and are always willing to help" (Year 2, student nurse),whilst also beginning to delegate to the HCAs. Both the HCA and student focus groups highlighted this relationship change occurred in Year 2 of the nurse degree but this was also at the point where student nurses generally worked less with HCAs."Helpful to work with HCA to a point, then it's restrictive . . . you will stop gaining knowledge at a point" (Year 2, student nurse).

The Year 3 students worked consistently with HCAs and reflected a more collaborative approach to service user care. Whilst mentors were "obeyed" (Year 3, student nurse), there was discussion, problem-solving, and joint decision-making with

Table 2.1 The four data themes.

The themes	Theme content
1. Roles and relationships	How students and HCAs develop an understanding or each other's roles in practice
2. Accessibility	How students engage with HCA for support and learning
3. Feedback	The acknowledgement of the HCAs contribution to learner feedback
4. Experience	How HCAs and learners value working and learning together to develop skills and knowledge in practice

HCAs."They [the HCA] want to make sure they teach you but in a different way and a different style" (Year 3, student nurse).

These findings reflect the well-established and much described hierarchy which is evident within the nursing profession (Morrow, Gustavson, and Jones, 2016) that can be prohibitive to learning skills such as critical thinking. A liminal state in Year 2 learners has been observed in other student cohorts (Zaitseva et al., 2013).

The findings suggest that for some students who have worked as HCAs previously, this unstable positioning, on the one hand valuing the Year 1 programme, but wanting to transition into the nursing profession may occur earlier in their education. Molesworth (2017) and Morley (2016) have previously identified the student journey to negotiate entry into the nursing community of practice.

2. Accessibility

The accessibility of the HCA is multifaceted; they can be in close physical proximity, emotionally available to nurture and look after the learner and practically more available to the student. "They are drawn more to the HCA because we sort of nurture them" (HCA) which, in turn, has an effect on learning; "I want to make them feel comfortable, which makes it easier for them to ask questions" (HCA). These statements were mirrored by the learners, who also commented that as the HCAs were not "signing my book" they were perceived as less threatening.

Most students worked with HCAs throughout their education, though how this occurred varied. It could be initiated by the learners, the HCA or the registered nurse, and could be purposeful or opportunistic. Several of the students had previously worked as an HCA, and thus were already partially acculturated to the group. The learners and HCAs both identified that not every HCA is well positioned to support a nursing student: "If the staff nurse gives the student to an HCA that isn't knowledgeable, then they won't learn" (HCA), and the learners agreed, wanting to be placed with someone who could support their learning. A willingness to engage with the students' learning needs was recognised as important by all groups.

3. Experience

Learners and HCAs identified clinical skills that were practiced together (Table 2.2). The HCAs felt that learners were more likely to approach an HCA to teach them certain skills due to feeling more comfortable to ask. Learners reported understanding the importance of working in team and felt that HCAs are part of the team when they are engaging. "I enjoy working with the HCA it helps us as students become better nurses" (Year 1, student nurse).

However, students have also experienced being spoken down to by HCAs. Individual experiences seemed to vary depending on the attitudes of the HCA and the student who "thinks they know it all" (HCA) and how they understand each other's roles.

As identified in Table 2.2, Year 1 learners observed the HCAs undertook the fundamental aspects of care and identified learning skills from the HCA. The students discussed the knowledge that the HCAs have in the general working environment, for example, knowing where things are kept if needed quickly. However, a Year 1 learner (with HCA experience) commented, "I've finished with . . . all these basic things so I feel that I want to work more with the nurses" (Year 1, student nurse).

Table 2.2 The clinical skills undertaken with HCAs, as reported by the students during their course.

Year 1	Year 2	Year 3
Monitoring vital signs	Refresh of existing skills	Refresh of existing skills
Urinalysis		Problem-solving
Documentation of observations		Communication
Nutritional need		Team-working
Elimination needs		
Pressure area care		
ECG testing		
Helping patients to socialise		
Cardiac monitoring		
Capillary Blood Glucose		
monitoring		

Morley (2015) found that students were initially grateful to HCAs for their support, but if this delayed their advancement to working with a registered nurse, they became frustrated. Year 2 students were unable to identify any specific skills that HCAs were able to teach and share with them that would contribute towards their learning. One student identified the HCA as a useful resource to re-cap on previously learnt skills but learning became limited. "When it comes to observations . . . not all . . . are fully knowledgeable" (Year 2, student nurse).

Most Year 2 students discussed having progressed from the skills that could be taught by the HCA, and their need to work with a registered nurse to progress further and learn additional skills, for example medication, catheterisation, drainage. This was found to be in contrast with the views of mentors, who listed catheterisation as a skill that could be learnt from a healthcare assistant, suggesting that the student is not aware of the full range of skills undertaken by HCAs in that practice area.

Year 3 students referred to the skills that had been learnt earlier in their education, for example, making a bed, referring someone and "all the small stuff." Year 3 students identified that communication, team working and problem solving were all skills that could be learnt from working with the HCAs and valued the skills learnt in Year 1.

Year 3 students acknowledged that whilst HCAs may not have full rationale for specific nursing interventions, they demonstrated tacit knowledge (Polanyi, 1966) and knowledge of the organisational culture could be gained from working with this group. "They just know everything, they know it inside out . . . they know who you should get in touch with, who you need, who is going to help you . . . that knowledge is fantastic" (Year 3, student nurse).

In particular, Year 3 students were beginning to appreciate the importance of a collaborative approach to practice: "We need to be able to work in teams-not just with HCA but with patients and their families" (Year 3, student nurses). Year 3 learners placed greater emphasis and importance on their own personal and professional development, therefore taking a broader view of HCA support as part of their learning (Bosley and Dale, 2008).

HCAs recognised and enjoyed the fact that their experience, knowledge, and training helped to contribute towards learning as well as benefiting staff nurses new to the practice area. The HCAs identified their knowledge of the culture of the organisation and their communication skills as relevant experience they could share to benefit others.

Students identified there can be limitations in knowledge of the HCAs, such as the theoretical underpinning of an intervention. They also acknowledged that if this occurred in practice, they would write down the query and either discuss it further with the mentor, research the explanation themselves, or the HCA would ask the nurse, thus enabling both to learn. The students also identified that there are many HCAs who registered as nurses abroad, but who are not registered with the Nursing and Midwifery Council (NMC) and thus unable to practice in the UK.

4. Feedback

There was no consistent approach reported by learners or HCAs of how feedback was given and received. Some learners reported receiving verbal feedback immediately when working with the HCA and found this beneficial to their learning. Others felt excluded when they observed the HCA and mentor in discussion: "I really don't know what's going on . . . I wish they told me" (Year 1, student nurse). The opportunity for professional discussion was lost.

The learners all agreed that the receipt of feedback was valuable to their learning and knowing where to improve, and Year 2 students felt that the lack of feedback given to them by the HCAs may be a result of the HCA themselves not receiving feedback or acknowledgement from the nursing team: "Some of them are like nurses, so knowledgeable, but they aren't being told this or how well they are doing, just told what to do" (Year 2, student nurse).

This was echoed by the HCAs, who stressed that their contribution to the learning environment "[has] to be acknowledged . . . acknowledgment is so important" (HCA).

They perceived that the student will mirror the attitude of the registered nurse in relation to how the HCA is valued and reflected on the role modelling which occurs in practice.

Year 3 learners were unaware that the HCA could document feedback, some reported receiving timely verbal feedback from the HCA, others via the mentors. One student commented that they thought the mentor would not seek feedback from the HCA, only from registered nurses, relating it to what they described as "the hierarchy."

The HCAs reported mixed methods of providing feedback to the learner, some felt comfortable to provide verbal feedback to the learner, others would discuss it directly with the mentor. None of the HCAs who participated in this research provided documented feedback to learners and were not aware there was opportunity to do so. The HCAs perceived 'the book' as being something exclusively for the assessor. They felt that if the learner was aware that they would be receiving feedback from HCA or via the assessor it would add to the learning, "they will realise that need to . . . not just help us, but learn something as they go along" (HCA).

The HCAs acknowledged that on occasion they are in a better position than the mentor to provide an accurate assessment of the learner due to the time spent together and opportunity to observe practice which the mentor may miss. One HCA recalled how she had been asked by a member of staff for her opinion of a learner and how she "felt so good that she had been counted and acknowledged" (HCA).

Responses from the mentors were varied, some mentors reported that they always sought feedback from the HCA, others advised that it was a less formal process where feedback was only given or received if there were concerns raised about the students' capabilities. They acknowledged that some HCAs are more confident in providing feedback than others, however, they felt that HCAs should always be asked for their feedback to contribute to their assessment, stressing the importance of this to enhance a collaborative team approach.

Conclusion

The NMC Standards for pre-registration nurse student supervision and assessment (NMC, 2018a) have acknowledged the wider team approach to supporting learning in practice. The findings of this research support Sarre et al.'s (2018) assertion that HCAs are keen to be involved in practice learning and have a role to play as 'helpful others'. The relationship between HCA and students can be a vital part of the learning experience but is dependent on the learning roles being clearly defined and supported by the whole team at different stages of the students' development. Chapter 1 has already identified the essential role of HCAs in the induction of students into the placement setting. Further analysis of the data collected, at a greater level of granularity, could further reveal the nuances of this relationship based on the different levels of experience of the participant sample used.

It is not without concern, however, to have students being educated to a professional level by unregistered staff. There is a current risk that professional education could be eroded by an over reliance on unregistered workforce due their availability to support student nurses in the absence of busy supervisors. However, this study, like Hasson et al. (2012) and Hasson (2013), has identified the hidden role that HCAs play in the education of students and that, only by explicitly naming this role, can a whole team approach to supporting learners in practice be promoted and the safety of patients ensured. This research and others (Bungay et al., 2016; Hasson et al., 2012; Gillespie and Rivers, 2017; Morley 2018) found HCAs had an 'ad hoc' teaching presence depending on the relationship they had with a student's mentor and how much their own professional role is valued. Undervaluing the abilities of HCAs has a negative impact on how they feel about their role within the nursing team, as seen in this study, and can lead to disengagement and lack of interest in HCAs utilising their skills and knowledge to support learners in practice (Willis, 2015).

The registered nurse needs to use clinical discernment and leadership skills to delegate learning to a team member who is prepared and knowledgeable, whilst retaining accountability for practice. As nurses feel they lack preparation in skills such as communication, professionalism, and leadership (Liebrecht and Montenery, 2016) it is vital that the importance and relevance of these skills are introduced to the students early in their education and identified as learning opportunities during their clinical experiences. The transition of the working and learning relationship between the student and HCA, identified in this study, could be a means by which this could be achieved.

Overall, the study has identified the need for a change in learning culture on placement where support roles for students are carefully examined and implemented from existing resources. A consistent approach to educating both HCAs and students to understand and value each other roles could potentially reduce traditional power differences and see greater long-term team centred professional growth. In practice it takes positive role-modelling by the registered nurse to support HCAs and students to facilitate and enable all to reflect on their collaborative learning (Padfield and Knowles, 2014).

Currently opportunities exist for HCAs and students to grow together as health care professionals. Professional development does not take place in isolation. The Care

Certificate standards can be mapped to NMC standards for Year 1 learners and the evolving nursing associate role to promote core values as the cornerstone of patient safety and the delivery of quality care (NMC, 2018b). Recognition of these opportunities are increasingly important with new routes into the nursing profession, such as the nursing associates and degree apprentices, who have to manage their dual roles of learner and employee.

With the HCAs required to undertake the Care Certificate and the formal registration of the nursing associates with the NMC, both groups need to meet specific standards with their skills, knowledge, and behaviour assessed. This includes receiving feedback and may result in these staff becoming more practiced in contributing to constructive feedback to others. The benefits to the learners in receiving feedback from all members of the team, including the HCA was been highlighted through the findings. As registered nurses are required to gain feedback from a variety of sources to meet their requirements for revalidation (NMC, 2018b), it is vital that student nurses are adequately prepared to seek, utilise, and reflect on feedback during their training, and requisite skills are nurtured and developed (Adamson et al., 2018). This research identified there is a change in relationship between the HCAs and learners as their educational programme progresses. This needs to be explored in more depth to ensure the changing dynamics and support needs are recognised and managed at all stages of the learners' journey, including HCA preparation for this transition.

Recommendations

1. Promote a team based, collaborative learning environment

To promote a positive and collaborative learning environment, it is important to involve the whole team and value the contributions that each member can make to support learners. This support can be from suitable 'helpful others', such as HCAs, who should be acknowledged and supervised in their support of students. With an evolving workforce, registered nurses will continue to be pivotal in bringing all learners together. These opportunities transcend nursing and include a more integrated culture of learning, as referred to in the NMC (2018a) standards.

2. Ensure students understand the scope of different roles in practice

In order to effectively work together, students and clinical staff need to understand each other's roles and scope of practice. This clarity is needed from day one in a practice area. This will help to manage expectations and best utilise scarce resources, as well as maximise learning. Chapter 1, 'Comprehensive orientation and socialisation,' recommends that each practice setting, in conjunction with their academic colleagues, provide key contact information, the profile of placement and the structure of clinical team, appropriate to a student's individual and programme orientation.

3. Promote a practice culture that values feedback and reflection as part of professional practice

Feedback and reflection is not an isolated experience but needs to be embedded in the whole culture to promote safe and effective practice for every member of the team and meet standards for revalidation. The practice supervisor and assessor roles promote feedback and role model different teaching styles at all levels, aspiring towards improving practice.

Case study for 'Helpful others': Recognising support networks for students in the clinical setting

Chapter 2 explores a team-based approach to learning and specifically the role of non-nurse trained care assistants in supporting practice learning. This case study highlights how this group of staff can support learning.

Jo is a student nurse on her final placement before qualification. Her practice assessor discusses with Jo the need to focus on her delegation skills and management of the ward in preparation for joining the NMC register. Jo is asked to reflect on her relationship with the health care assistants and consider how she will further develop her leadership skills.

What is the learning aim?

To support Jo to consider the role of the healthcare assistant and how she can enhance her learning by working with the whole team.

What learning will be achieved?

1   To assist Jo to connect and recognise her developing relationship with health care assistants as she approaches registration
2   To establish the roles and responsibilities of the clinical team to aide Jo in her delegation and leadership decisions.
3   To expand Jo's knowledge of the responsibilities and accountabilities of the registered nurse and their practical application.

How can learning be supported?

1. To encourage Jo to reflect on how her practice has been informed by her time working with the health care assistants. This will include the value placed on this role within a whole team approach to care.

Padfield and Knowles (2014) identified a range of tacit learning opportunities (Polanyi, 1966) which students experience when working with health care assistants throughout their education. This is often not explicitly acknowledged, and students need support to recognise the how this learning occurs, which may differ from the formal education undertaken with a nurse (Hasson et al., 2012).

2. To effectively and safely delegate care in the practice environment, it is first necessary for Jo to establish an understanding of the roles and responsibilities of each member of the team, as well as their practical competencies and limitations.

Many HCAs have numerous and extended roles within practice areas. To demonstrate safe leadership, a good knowledge of the range of skills undertaken and by whom needs to be established. New workers and students in practice areas need time to develop this understanding. This will include considering the clinical interventions which require further training. With the expansion of the nursing profession to include the nursing associates with their clinical competency range, teams will need to consider the roles in their own practice environments and how professional and personal development can be achieved for all.

3. To expand and develop leadership skills, Jo will need to understand and effectively apply her knowledge of The Code (NMC, 2018b) in regard to her responsibilities and accountabilities.

The NMC (2018b) code of conduct is clear: registered nurses are accountable for the care which occurs in their practice area. It is imperative that students are better prepared for delegation during their pre-registration education (Liebrecht and Montenery, 2016). The experience of working with healthcare assistants can support a better understanding of the roles and effective communication strategies. This needs to be role modelled in practice by the registered nurses and students given opportunity to enhance and expand these skills under supervision.

References

Adamson, E., King, L., Foy, L., McLeod, M., Traynor, J., Watson, W. and Gray, M. (2018) Feedback in clinical practice: Enhancing the students' experience through action research *Nurse Education in Practice*, 31, pp. 48–53.

Annear, M., Lea, E. and Robinson, A. (2014) Are care workers appropriate mentors for nursing students in residential aged care? *BMC Nursing*, 13(1), pp. 44–48.

Bazian. (2016) RCN mentorship project 2015. From today's support in practice to tomorrow's vision for excellence. *Royal College of Nursing*. Available at: https://www.rcn.org.uk/professiona l-development/publications/pub-005454 (accessed 10/8/18).

Bisholt, B., Ohlsson, U., Engström, A.K., Johansson, A.S., and Gustafsson, M. (2014) Nursing students' assessment of the learning environment in different clinical settings. *Nurse Education in Practice*, 14(1), pp. 304–310.

Bosley, S. and Dale, J. (2008) Healthcare assistants in general practice: Practical and conceptual issues of skill-mix change. *British Journal of General Practice*, 58(547), pp. 118–124.

Bungay, H., Jackson, J. and Lord, S. (2016) Exploring assistant practitioners' views of their role and training. *Nursing Standard*, 30(30), pp. 46–52.

Burrow, M., Gilmour, J. and Cook, C. (2017) Healthcare assistants and aged residential care: A challenging policy and contractual environment. *Nursing Praxis in New Zealand; Palmerston North*, 33(2), pp. 7–19.

Cavendish, C. (2013) The Cavendish Review: An independent review into healthcare assistants and support workers in the NHS and social care settings. Available at: https://www.gov.uk/ government/publications/review-of-healthcare-assistants-and-support-workers-in-nhs-and-socia l-care (accessed 11/21/18).

Clarke, P. (2015) Student nurses on placement – collaborators or challengers. *The Journal of Adult Protection*, 17(5), pp. 287–295.

Eraut, M. (2007) Learning from other people in the workplace. *Oxford Review of Education*, 33(4), pp. 403–422.

Gillespie, M. and Rivers, I. (2017) Assistant grade nurses and nursing students: A diary study. *Mental Health Practice*, 21(3), pp. 21–25.

Gray, M.A. and Smith, L.N. (2000) The qualities of an effective mentor from the student nurse's perspective: Findings from a longitudinal qualitative study. *Journal of Advanced Nursing*, 32(6), pp. 1542–1549.

Hasson, F. (2013) Delegating and supervising the unregistered professionals: The student nurse experience. *Nurse Education Today*, 33(3), pp. 229–235.

Hasson, F., McKenna, H. and Keeney, S. (2012) Perceptions of the unregistered healthcare worker's role in pre-registration student nurses' clinical training. *Journal of Advanced Nursing*, 69(7), pp. 1618–1629.

Johnson, M., Magnusson, C., Allan, H., Evans, K., Ball, E., Horton, K., Curtis, K. and Westwood, S. (2015) 'Doing the writing' and 'working in parallel': How 'distal nursing' affects delegation and supervision in the emerging role of the newly qualified nurse. *Nurse Education Today*, 35(2), pp. 29–33.

Liebrecht, C. and Montenery, S. (2016) Use of simulated psychosocial role-playing to enhance nursing students' development of soft skills. *Creative Nursing; Minneapolis*, 22(3), pp. 171–175.

Molesworth, M. (2017) Nursing students' first placement: Peripherality and marginality within the community of practice. *Journal of Nursing Education*, 56(1), pp. 31–38.

Morley, D.A. (2015) A grounded theory study exploring first year student nurses' learning in practice, (Doctor in Professional Practice thesis), Bournemouth University, Bournemouth.

Morley, D. (2016) Applying Wenger's communities of practice theory to placement learning. *Nurse Education Today*, 39, pp. 161–162.

Morley, D. (2018) The 'ebb and flow' of student learning on placement. In Morley, D. (ed), *Enhancing employability in higher education through work-based learning*. Switzerland: Palgrave Macmillan, pp. 173–190.

Morrow, K., Gustavson, A. and Jones, J. (2016) Speaking Up behaviours (safety voices) of healthcare workers: A meta-synthesis of qualitative research studies. *International Journal of Nursing Studies*, 64, pp. 42–51.

Myall, M., Levett-Jones, T. and Lathlean, J. (2008) Mentorship in contemporary practice: the experiences of nursing students and practice mentors. *Journal of Clinical Nursing*, 17(1), pp. 834–842.

NHS Digital. (2018) NHS workforce statistics. Available at: https://digital.nhs.uk/data-and-in formation/publications/statistical/nhs-workforce-statistics/nhs-workforce-statistics-novem ber-2017-provisional-statistics#resources (accessed 10/19/18).

Nursing and Midwifery Council (NMC). (2018a) Standards for nurses: Standards for student supervision and assessment. Available at: https://www.nmc.org.uk/standards-for-education-a nd-training/standards-for-student-supervision-and-assessment/ (accessed on 06/21/18).

Nursing and Midwifery Council (NMC). (2018b) The code: Professional standards of practice and behaviour for nurses, midwives and nursing associates. Available at: https://www.nmc.org.uk/sta ndards/code/ (accessed 10/19/18).

O'Driscoll, M., Allan, H. and Smith, P. (2010) Still looking for leadership – Who is responsible for student nurses' learning in practice? *Nurse Education Today*, 30(3), pp. 212–217.

Padfield, B. and Knowles, R. (2014) Development of learning facilitation roles for unregistered practitioners. *Nursing Standard*, 29(16), pp. 16–18.

Polanyi, M. (1966) *The tacit dimension*. London: Routledge and Kegan Paul.

Sarre, S., Maben, J., Aldus, C., Schneider, J., Wharrad, H., Nicholson, C. and Arthur, A. (2018) The challenges of training, support and assessment of healthcare support workers: A qualitative study of experiences in three English acute hospitals. *International Journal of Nursing Studies*, 79, pp.145–153.

Thornley, C. (2000) A question of competence? Re-evaluating the roles of the nursing auxiliary and health care assistant in the NHS. *Journal of Clinical Nursing*, 9(3), pp. 451–458.

Traverse. (2018) *Evaluation of introduction of Nursing Associates: Phase 1 report*. Health Education England. Available at: https://www.hee.nhs.uk/sites/default/files/documents/Phase%201% 20OPM%20Evaluation%20Report%20%28002%29.pdf (accessed 03/15/19).

Unison. (2010) Developing high performance support workforce in acute healthcare settings. Oxford University. Available at: https://www.sbs.ox.ac.uk/faculty-research/health-care/resea

rch/support-worker-research/developing-high-performance-support-workforce-acute-healthca re-setting (accessed 06/21/18).

Willis, P. (2015) Raising the bar. Shape of Caring: A review of the future education and training of registered nurses and care assistants. *Health Education England.* Available at: https://www.hee. nhs.uk/sites/default/files/documents/2348-Shape-of-caring-review-FINAL.pdf (accessed 06/ 21/18).

Zaitseva, E., Milsom, C. and Stewart, M. (2013) Connecting the dots: Using concept maps for interpreting student satisfaction. *Quality in Higher Education*, 19(2), pp. 225–247.

3 Student peer support and learning

Kathy Wilson (k.wilson@mdx.ac.uk), Nora Cooper and Maurina Baron

Introduction

Chapter 3 explores the potential value of peer support and learning which has been described as 'gaining momentum as a global phenomenon' (Keenan, 2014, p. 5). With the reported benefits for improving student satisfaction, retention and employability skills this expansion is attributed in the main to the increased focus on enhancing the student experience in higher education (Hilsdon, 2014; Keenan, 2014).

Peer learning has been defined as 'reciprocal learning activities' (Boud, Cohen and Sampson, 2001, p. 5) involving students learning collaboratively in a variety of ways and whilst there are several terms associated with peer learning and support that are often interchangeable (Brannagan et al., 2013). In the nursing and midwifery literature, peer-mentoring is the most common term used (Jacobs, 2017; Rohatinsky, Harding and Carriere, 2017) whilst peer-assisted learning (PAL) and peer-assisted study sessions (PASS) are more common across a broader range of disciplines in UK Higher Education (Keenan, 2014). With the publication of the NMC standards for education and training it seems timely to revisit the value of peer led approaches and create a much-needed critical dialogue regarding its implementation to support the education of the future workforce (NMC, 2018).

Within this chapter a qualitative methodology has been utilised to explore nursing and midwifery students' experience and perceptions of peer learning and support in practice. Currently there is a paucity of published empirical studies reflecting a UK perspective focusing on practice settings (Jacobs, 2017; Rohatinsky et al., 2017; HEE, 2018).

Literature Review

Why is there an increasing focus on peer learning in nursing and midwifery education?

The NMC (NMC, 2018) standards framework for nursing and midwifery education stipulate the need to 'empower and support students to become resilient, caring, reflective and lifelong learners' (p. 10) proposing that they should 'have opportunities to learn with and from peers' (p. 11). The need for nursing students to acquire enhanced leadership and supervision skills (NMC, 2018) further reinforces the need for alternative pedagogies such as peer learning.

Within nursing and midwifery education there is extensive literature extolling the benefits of peer support and learning approaches at different stages of the students' professional journey (Aston and Molassiotis, 2003; Sprengel and Job, 2004; Dennison, 2010;

Brannagan et al., 2013; Morley, 2015). A number of organisations world-wide have introduced peer support as part of their recruitment strategy, in some instances successfully targeting community groups who may not have traditionally studied nursing or midwifery (Smith, Beattie and Kyle, 2015). Examples include supporting Year 1 students with transition and socialisation (Loke and Chow, 2007; Harmer et al., 2011; McKeller and Kempster, 2017), peer tutoring to support academic development and both peer review and peer assessment within the clinical laboratory and practice setting (Godson, Wilson and Goodman, 2007; Dennison, 2010; Brannagan et al., 2013; Won and Choi, 2017).

Bagnardi (2011, p. 37) explains the need for a peer mentoring initiative around 'faculty shortages', a perspective reflected in a number of studies from the US (Rohatinsky et al., 2017). Dennison (2010) also claims that peer mentoring programmes may be a solution to lessening the burden on teaching staff. This supplemental approach however is criticised by Hilsdon (2014) for representing more of a deficit model rather than a learning development approach.

2. What is the relevance of peer learning to practice education?

The importance of effective staff-student relationships and student supervision are viewed as key in creating a positive learning environment (Papastavrou et al., 2010; Newton et al., 2014). Students often report feeling overwhelmed due to poor staffing issues and regularly report that their learning is not prioritised (HEE, 2018). They need to feel appreciated, recognised as part of the team and actively engaged in their learning (Papp, Markkanen and von Bonsdorff, 2003; Horsfall et al., 2012; Newton et al., 2014). Creating this important sense of belongingness is well documented in the literature (Bradbury-Jones, Sambrook and Irvine, 2010; Levett-Jones and Lathlean, 2008; Morley, 2015) and is an aspect of practice where the benefits of peer support have been shown to be most effective. The CLiP model, critiqued further in Chapter 5 on expansive learning, emphasises peer support in practice as part of the team approach to coaching (Clarke, Williamson and Kane, 2018).

The main practice-based approaches documented from outside the UK vary in purpose and length and so make it difficult to draw conclusions. Studies from the United States describe peer support models ranging from two hours to two days that mainly focus on the initial orientation to a new area (Rohatinsky et al., 2017). Examples from Sweden provide an evaluation of models over a two-week period with reports of students developing independence and taking more responsibility for their own learning despite this short period of time (Hellström-Hyson, Mårtensson and Kristofferzon, 2011; Pålsson et al., 2014; Lofmark and Wikblad, 2001; Secomb, 2008).

Christiansen and Bell (2007) reviewed the experience of students in the UK who reportedly engaged in peer relationships naturally in practice. Aston and Molassiotis (2003) provides one of the few UK examples of an empirical study capturing the supervision and support experiences of 31 senior students and 27 junior students during their clinical placement. Other examples refer to the peer relationship as Dyads where students are paired with each other or a Coach and Buddy System for students (CABSS) (Baker and Sheehy, 2017).

It could be argued that the reassurance experienced by peers will not only help sustain students during difficult times (Aston and Molassiotis, 2003) but also support in developing their resilience (Killingley, 2016) resulting in enhanced student experiences and improved retention (HEE, 2018).

3. What needs to be considered to ensure effective implementation of peer learning?

Within the reviewed literature several benefits are highlighted related to socialisation, increased learning, enhanced communication, leadership skills and improved personal growth (Jacobs, 2017; Christiansen and Bell, 2010). Rohatinsky et al. (2017), however, believe that further evaluation needs to be undertaken to support the validity and credibility of these approaches.

The challenges expressed by senior students need to be considered to enhance the potential success of peer strategies. Students reported becoming frustrated when their peers did not prepare in advance of a session or they turned up late for the sessions as part of a peer tutoring scheme (Won and Choi, 2017). A number also reported feeling under pressure because of other time commitments, doubting their own level of knowledge and finding managing differences in personalities and learning styles challenging (Loke and Chow, 2007; Won and Choi, 2017).

For many authors the key areas that required attention to ensure effective and successful implementation were related to issues of preparation, understanding expectations, gaining support for the role and receiving feedback (Aston and Molassiotis, 2003; Colvin and Ashman, 2010; Brannagan et al., 2013). Keenan (2014) purports that peer learning needs to be embedded more widely and may require cultural transformations at both the level of pedagogy and institutional practice.

Methodology

The motivation to undertake this project stemmed from a critical evaluation of a learning and teaching strategy introduced in March–May 2017 in which a group of 14 Year 3 nursing students in their final placement were invited to be a peer mentor for a Year 1 student nurse within the clinical area. The preparation was undertaken electronically and open communications maintained via email and face to face meetings with both sets of students. The educational teams and link lecturers in the organisations were also involved and provided ad hoc support. Students were encouraged to raise issues, provide ongoing feedback and were invited to undertake an online evaluation at the end of the placement period. Whilst there were some benefits identified from the feedback, only 28 per cent of the Year 3 students felt that this was a positive initiative and cited multiple factors for this. It was therefore proposed that further research in this area was needed to gain a better understanding of the student perspective to support peer development for future curricula.

Ethical approval was granted from the University's Ethics Committee. This study used a qualitative methodology to develop an in-depth understanding of the nursing and midwifery students' perspectives of their peer learning and mentoring in practice. There were two key stages: Stage 1, in May 2018, involved focus groups with Year 3 students in their final placement (n= 18) and Stage 2 in June 2018 involved focus groups with a group of midwifery students (n=7) who had been supported in acute adult ward areas by a group of nursing students (n=5).

Stage 1 of the research

Two groups of Year 3 final placement students were invited to participate in a discussion regarding peer support and learning. Students were fully informed of the purpose of the research and confirmed their agreement to participate through completion of the project consent forms. Four key questions were posed and students were invited to respond.

1   Have you had experience of providing support and guiding peers with their learning in practice?
2   What would you consider are the benefits for senior learners and for junior learners?
3   What do you perceive to be the challenges?
4   In what way has your programme prepared you for this?

Results

Question 1: Have you had experience of providing support and guiding peers with their learning in practice?

Most of the senior group of students indicated that they had some experience of supporting junior learners though this was something they initiated: "This is something we just do anyway" (Year 3, adult nurse student). In the main, examples reflected support for Year 1 students to help them settle into the ward as third years remembered it being challenging. One student reported: "It's easier talking to another student and I always look out for Year 1 student because I remember how difficult it was when I started" (Year 3, adult nurse student).

Overall some students wanted to offer regular peer support despite the challenges with shift allocations which made it difficult to connect with junior students.

Question 2: What would you consider are the benefits of peer support and learning for you as senior learners and for junior learners?

The benefits of peer support to a junior student were highlighted particularly in relation to helping them settle into the placement and having someone to pose questions to.

"I remember as a new student being really grateful to a Year 2 student who helped explain some of the terminology after the morning report and I felt I could always go to her" (Year 3, adult nurse student).

Students also articulated some of the benefits to themselves as senior students and acknowledged that reciprocal learning is "a really good idea as we can both learn from each other, they can learn from me and they might also teach me something" (Year 3, adult nurse student). One student specifically related this to her future mentor role: "As a senior learner I can see that it helps us gain experience of teaching and so better prepares us for qualifying and it encourages junior students to settle and learn" (Year 3, adult nurse student).

One of the Year 3 students reported that she had been asked to speak to the Year 2 group as part of their preparation for practice and was very willing and proud to take on this role. What was clear from this discussion was that students becoming involved for shorter periods of time, and having access to do so, benefitted both groups of students.

Question 3: What do you perceive to be the challenges?

This question appeared to engage a group of students that had offered little to the discussion up until this point. Some seemed anxious about teaching junior students, even though they were close to registration. One student raised concerns that a Year 3 student might not have sufficient knowledge to teach another student as "not all students like to teach" (Year 3, adult nurse student).

Further concerns raised by students were linked to workload and staffing issues as well as accountability. Whilst the Year 3 student nurses remain supernumerary during their final placement experience, they were likely to take on additional responsibilities under more indirect supervision and so, at times, could feel unsupported in their own learning.

"There are no benefits to undertake this role that I can see as we are already so busy and don't even get to spend enough time with our mentors . . . it's an added pressure and time is a problem as we are not always treated as supernumerary" (Year 3, adult nurse student).

Question 4: In what way has your programme prepared you to support peers in practice?

When asked if students had any preparation in their programme related to teaching and learning most students indicated that this was either limited or non-existent. Two child health students described a model whereby they teach Year 2 students in the skills laboratory as part of their module assessment and had a period of preparation prior to the sessions. "We were given preparation by teaching Year 2 students a skill in the skills lab as part of our Year 3 assessment which was really good" (Year 3, child health student). The other students responded positively to this example and demonstrated an appetite to work collegiately and collaboratively to expand their learning.

Stage 2 of the research

A discussion within one of our local placement organisations highlighted the challenges that some Year 2 midwifery students have during a two-week adult care experience out of their midwifery experience. This was due mainly to the unfamiliarity of the environment and concerns regarding unrealistic expectations of mentors during a two-week period. The project team felt that this was an opportunity to enhance support for these midwifery students with the introduction of a peer model involving the student nurses already allocated to those areas. This midwifery student group was anxious about their nursing placement and the team felt it could benefit both groups of students and potentially further enhance our understanding of utilising different peer support and learning approaches.

Midwifery students (n=7) were allocated to senior nursing students in acute medical/surgical areas across two placement organisations via purposive sample. The main aim was to provide support, similar to a buddy system for the length of the placement and to also review potential benefits and challenges for both groups of participants. The student nurses were initially contacted by email to explain the project to them and allow them the opportunity to ask any questions. The students that did respond were also invited to participate and the overwhelmingly positive response reflected the enthusiasm and motivation of this group of senior nursing students.

The midwifery students were invited to a workshop in preparation for practice where interested students, provided their consent to participate. Information about the initiative was also sent to practice placement staff who supported students to elicit their support and all reported that they were happy to be involved. Following the two-week placement a focus group was held with the midwifery students when they returned to university. The five nursing students all provided feedback via email. The following questions were posed, with question 2 not applicable to the nursing students:

1   Did you get to meet your buddy/student in the first two days?
2   How supported did you feel?

3   What do you think were the benefits for you?
4   How do you think the experience could be improved?

Results

Feedback from the nurse students was invited via email as they were still on placement. From the thematic analysis of all of the feedback three key themes were identified.

1 Being welcoming and supportive

Whilst this was a short placement experience, most the midwifery students felt that their overall experience had been enhanced by the identification of a student nurse peer. Student midwives particularly appreciated meeting their peer on the first day of placement.

Within the focus group there was a sense of being able to ask questions of their 'buddy' that they could not ask the registered nurse.

"As a student I felt more comfortable with another student and far more free to communicate and ask questions and not feel embarrassed and there was no judgement from her" (Year 2, student midwife).

Feedback from nursing students was also largely positive and were able to recognise the benefits to the midwifery students in particular,

> I feel it made the student less anxious and having a friendly face to welcome them to a new environment helps especially as it's a speciality out of their comfort zone and branch of expertise. It also helps with their communication skills for new teams and introductions.
>
> (Year 3, adult nurse student)

This experience would have been more positive had off duties been matched more closely.

It seemed that for midwifery students in a nursing environment the positive impact was even more evident. The mutual benefits here also extended to understanding the roles of students in different professional groups.

2 Positive Role Modelling

Whilst the nursing students did not teach any specific skills they were asked to guide the midwifery students and help them to gain the support they might need.

> As I am a final year student on my sign off placement I was able to use part of this experience to build interpersonal and professional skills into what mentoring is about and how I would facilitate my prospective student when I become a staff nurse.
>
> (Year 3, adult nurse student)

The midwifery students admired the knowledge and skills shown by the nursing students, with one student stating she wanted to be like her buddy as she felt very supported. "I see her as a great role model and hope I can be like her someday" (Year 2, student midwife).

3 Wider communication issues in the practice context

Whilst support from ward managers and placement facilitators was sought prior to the initiative, two nursing students reported that they had not been allowed to have their roster planned to meet the midwifery student on day one and this was disappointing for both groups. Where two of the senior students did try to intervene to manage their role in line with the midwifery students they were challenged by staff members who were unaware of the arrangements and so were unwilling to alter the students' rotas.

One of the drawbacks of pairing the midwifery students with a senior nursing student was the fact that a formal mentorship model was not always arranged for the midwifery student as this was viewed as the responsibility of the Year 3 student nurse.

Analysis

Despite the limitations of the size of the study, the findings aid the understanding of the positive potential that peer support and learning models offer. For the recipient of peer support, in this case the Year 2 student midwives, it encouraged the students not only to settle and learn but also feel acknowledged and validated, as found by Glass and Walter (2000). It was also found to reduce anxiety in an unfamiliar setting (Kleehammer, Hart and Keck, 1990; Shipton, 2002; Sprengel and Job, 2004; Walker and Verklan, 2016).

For the Year 3 adult nursing students who were facilitating the peer support, there was evidence of both intrinsic and extrinsic advantages. It offered the opportunity for students to reflect on their own practice, bringing new insights and enhanced understanding gained from that experience. These findings concur with Bagnardi (2011) and Fisher and Stanyer (2018). Many authors have discussed the value of peer approaches to develop confidence, self-management, leadership, problem solving skills and emotional intelligence (Christiansen and Bell, 2010; Jacobs, 2017; Rohatinsky et al., 2017) as well as complementary self-awareness and self-regulation in preparation for professional roles (Won and Choi, 2017; Dennison, 2010; Fisher and Stanyer, 2018). Enabling students to provide constructive feedback is also essential to their future roles (Rohatinsky et al., 2017; NMC, 2018) although this was not commented upon by the students in this study.

Students who participated as part of the focus group alluded to barriers and challenges; however, many of the students in the focus group had not been in a position of being the 'follower', a role in which students can learn to be the 'leader' through reflection and self-growth. Those senior students who had experience of supporting the learning of junior colleagues could recognise the consolidation of their own knowledge and skills and this supports Christiansen and Bell's (2010) findings where the senior student often reports deeper learning and understanding.

Students experienced barriers created by members of the team in practice which impacted on identifying time to spend with their allocated peer. Colvin and Ashman (2010) emphasise the importance of being aware of the potential for resistance and resultant issues of power. Some students also felt frustrated that there was often lack of recognition of their own learning needs and that they were left to support the junior peer who subsequently did not benefit from formal supervision. As a result, there was a risk that the learning needs of both parties could be ignored (Christiansen and Bell, 2010). These additional responsibilities created unwanted pressures leaving the Year 3 students feeling frustrated as, at times, they were left to fill the gap.

Conclusion

Peer learning approaches have been introduced widely in response to calls to improve student retention, engagement and success (Hilsdon, 2014). This applies to both nursing and midwifery programmes and with the changes to the education standards for pre-registration nursing and midwifery in the UK (NMC, 2018) the potential benefits of implementing peer support and learning models needs to be explored and formally evaluated beyond the research presented in this chapter.

Findings from this study reflect the published research in terms of perceived benefits as well as some of the barriers and challenges. An effective peer relationship can add to a sense of belonging, promote cooperative learning and support enhanced employability skills enabling and supporting students to take a more proactive role in their learning and the learning of others (NMC, 2018). It is acknowledged that a longitudinal study of peer support, using a larger sample of students, would have a greater chance of isolating more specific areas of student development. The study also begins to highlight power differentials of peer support against the support of registered staff, necessitating the clarity and consensus of roles amongst learners and supervisors suggested by Aston and Molassiotis (2003) and Hilsdon (2014).

Whilst some have identified the cost effectiveness of peer support (Dennison, 2010), and its potential to reduce staff burden and increase student numbers in placement, peer approaches should be introduced for their potential strengths for learning and not primarily for building capacity and addressing staff shortages (Rohatinsky et al., 2017). The literature review for Chapter 5 highlights some early criticism of the CLiP project for its potential overreliance on peer support.

Overall, this chapter argues that peer learning can contribute to student learning in a variety of positive ways though careful preparation, time to undertake the role, realistic expectations and a supportive learning culture to ensure effective and safe implementation (NMC, 2018). It is essential that managers, programme teams, students and practice staff do not underestimate the work needed to embed this approach within the placement culture and are open to fully explore the potential barriers as well as the benefits. Peer learning and support should be realised for its excellent potential in enhancing practice learning and contributing to positive student experiences as part of a team-based approach which Morley, Wilson and McDermott (2017) propose as part of a more rounded model of practice learning.

Recommendations

1. Embed peer support and learning in practice

Peer learning models need to be explicitly explored and embedded as a valuable, alternative pedagogical approach within curriculum delivery and the area of practice learning. There is the potential that students, who themselves experience the benefits of having a peer from Year 1, will value the approach and take on the responsibility more readily as they progress through their programme. The student experiences need to be evaluated and their strategies built upon for the success of future peer learning development.

2. Introduce a diversity of approaches

A range of approaches could be staged along the student journey and involve both peer teaching and assessment initiatives. A framework, such as the coaching model developed as part of the expansive learning theme in Chapter 5, provides a structured and coherent approach where students adopt different roles based on the situation and peer need. Students need to be empowered through the development of their confidence and competence to move from a role as a buddy to that of a 'learning and coaching partner'.

3. Institutional Support and Preparation

Clarity regarding roles and expectations is critical. Students need to understand their levels of responsibility and accountability and have access to support as needed. Institutional support is essential so that sufficient time and resources are allocated to undertake the appropriate level of exploration, preparation, ongoing support and evaluation that is needed for effective implementation. Working in close partnership with placement organisations so that they are part of the development, implementation and evaluation of practice-based approached is crucial to its success.

Case Study for Student peer support and learning

This chapter presents peer support models where senior and junior students paired together in practice can work and learn collaboratively. This is specifically beneficial in enabling students to have more involvement in their learning (Clarke et al., 2018) promoting skills of self-direction and self-regulation. This case study outlines how two students can support each other in developing an understanding of their assessment to support their learning.

Keylai and Afua are Year 2 students who are anxious about their practice assessment document. They are both finding it challenging to meet with their supervisors in order to discuss the requirements and objectives set in their documents. The local practice facilitator suggests to them that they think of alternative ways of ensuring that their own learning. Keylai and Afua decided to find a quiet place to discuss and exchange views about their practice assessment requirements.

What is the learning aim?

To enable Keylai and Afua to better understand their own learning and assessment needs and to enable them to take more responsibility for their own learning and the learning of others.

What learning will be achieved?

1   To enable Keylai and Afua to share their understanding in a safe environment, ask questions and support each other.
2   To increase the assessment literacy of Keylai and Afua through enhanced understanding of assessment requirements.
3   To empower Keylai and Afua to take active roles in directing their own learning and the learning of others.

How can learning be supported?

1 To enable students to share their understanding in a safe environment, ask questions and support each other.

Keylai and Afua should feel safe to challenge each other's current knowledge regarding their understanding of the assessment requirement. In trying to solve novel problems, perceptual or conceptual similarities between existing shared knowledge (obtained from information given in the classroom) and a new problem (encountered in the practice area) can remind students of what they already know. In line with socio constructivist theory, Keylai and Afua must actively construct new information into their existing mental framework for meaningful learning to occur.

2 To increase assessment literacy through promoting enhanced understanding of assessment requirements

Assessment literacy 'involves a combination of knowledge, skills and competencies and equips individuals with an appreciation of the purpose and processes of assessment' (Price et al., 2012 p. 10). Assessment is viewed as a significant driver for student learning (Race, 2014) and hence it is important for students to understand and take responsibility and ownership of their own assessment. Working together and asking each other questions regarding specific standards or requirements Keylai and Afua can challenge each other's understanding and develop a deeper understanding of the assessment requirements.

3 To empower students to take active roles in directing their own learning and the learning of others

Enhancing an individuals' abilities to meet their own needs and solve their own problems is strongly linked with the concept of empowerment (Bradbury-Jones et al., 2010). Peer support plays a major role in empowering students and aiding in the facilitation of the learning opportunities they need in order to achieve the desired proficiencies for registration (NMC, 2018). By being given the time to undertake this peer review Keylai and Afua will feel valued in that their learning needs have been recognised and will have gained in confidence and become more assertive in engaging with their learning.

References

Aston, L. and Molassiotis, A. (2003) 'Supervising and supporting student nurses in clinical placements: The peer support initiative', *Nurse Education Today*, (23), pp. 202–210.

Baker, G. and Sheehy, K. (2017) 'The innovation of a fellowship role to promote mentor models in clinical practice for pre-registration nurses', *Health Education England*. Available at: https://www.heacademy.ac.uk/system/files/hub/download/d2st10s6_gillian_baker.pdf (accessed 03/12/18).

Bagnardi, M. (2011) 'Transitioning to practice: A nursing student peer mentoring leadership initiative', *I-manager's Journal on Nursing*, 1(3), pp. 37–42.

Boud, D., Cohen, R. and Sampson, J. (2001) *Peer learning in higher education: Learning from and with each other*. London: Kogan Page.

Brannagan, K.B., Dellinger, A., Thomas, J., Mitchell, D., Lewis-Trabeaux, S. and Dupre, S. (2013) 'Impact of peer teaching on nursing students: Perceptions of learning environment, self-efficacy, and knowledge', *Nurse Education Today*, 33(11), pp. 1440–1447.

Bradbury-Jones, C., Sambrook, S. and Irvine, I. (2010) 'Empowering and being valued: A phenomenological study of nursing students' experiences of clinical practice', *Nurse Education Today*, 31(4), pp. 368–372.

Christiansen, A. and Bell, A. (2010) 'Peer learning partnerships: Exploring the experience of pre-registration nursing students', *Journal of Clinical Nursing*, 19(5–6), pp. 803–810.

Clarke, D., Williamson, G.R. and Kane, A. (2018) 'Could students' experiences of clinical placements be enhanced by implementing a Collaborative Learning in Practice (CLiP) model?' *Nurse Education in Practice*, 33, pp. A3–A5.

Colvin, J.W. and Ashman, M. (2010) 'Roles, risks & resistance; Benefits of peer mentoring', *Relationships in Higher Education*, 18(2), pp. 121–134.

Dennison, S. (2010) 'Peer mentoring: Untapped potential', *The Journal of Nursing Education*, 49(6), pp. 340–342.

Fisher, M. and Stanyer, R. (2018) 'Peer mentoring: Enhancing the transition from student to professional', *Midwifery*, 60, pp. 56–59.

Glass, N. and Walter, R. (2000) 'An experience of peer mentoring with student nurses: Enhancement of personal and professional growth', *The Journal of Nursing Education*, 39(4), pp. 155–160.

Godson, N.R., Wilson, A. and Goodman, M. (2007) 'Evaluating student learning in the clinical skills laboratory', *British Journal of Nursing*, 16(15), pp. 942–945.

Harmer, B., Huffman, J., Johnson, B. (2011) Clinical peer mentoring: Partnering BSN seniors and sophomores on a dedicated education unit, *Nurse Educator*, 36(5) pp. 197–202.

Health Education England (HEE). (2018) RePAIR: Reducing pre-registration attrition and improving retention report. https://www.hee.nhs.uk/our-work/reducing-pre-registration-attrition-improving-retention (accessed 11/02/18).

Hellström-Hyson, E., Mårtensson, G. and Kristofferzon, M. (2012) 'To take responsibility or to be an onlooker: Nursing students' experiences of two models of supervision', *Nurse Education Today*, 32(1), pp. 105–110.

Hilsdon, J. (2014) 'Peer learning for change in higher education', *Innovations in Education and Teaching International*, 51(3), pp. 244–254.

Horsfall, J., Cleary, M. and Hunt, G. (2012) 'Developing a pedagogy for nursing teaching and learning', *Nurse Education Today*, 32(8), pp. 930–933.

Jacobs, S. (2017) 'A scoping review examining nursing student peer mentorship', *Journal of Professional Nursing*, 33(3), pp. 212–223.

Keenan, C. (2014) 'Mapping student-led peer learning in the UK', *The Higher Education Academy*. Available at: https://www.heacademy.ac.uk/system/files/resources/peer_led_learning_keenan_nov_14-final.pdf (accessed 06/20/18).

Killingley, J. (2016) 'Thinking outside the box', *Midwives*, 19, pp. 72–73.

Kleehammer, K., Hart, A.L. and Keck, J.F. (1990) 'Nursing students' perceptions of anxiety producing situations in the clinical setting', *Journal of Nursing Education*, 29(4), pp. 183–187.

Levett-Jones, T. and Lathlean, J. (2008) 'Belongingness: A prerequisite for nursing students' clinical learning', *Nurse Education in Practice*, 8(2), pp. 103–111.

Lofmark, A. and Wikblad, K. (2001) 'Facilitating and obstructing factors for development of learning in clinical practice: A student perspective', *Journal of Advanced Nursing*, 34(1), pp. 43–50.

Loke, A.J.T. and Chow, F.L.W. (2007) 'Learning partnership-the experience of peer tutoring among nursing students: A qualitative study', *International Journal of Nursing Studies*, 44(2), pp. 237–244.

McKellar, L. and Kempster, C. (2017) 'We're all in this together: Midwifery student peer mentoring', *Nurse Education in Practice*, 24, pp. 112–117.

Morley, D. A. (2015) A grounded theory study exploring first year student nurses' learning in practice. Doctor in Professional Practice thesis. Bournemouth, UK: Bournemouth University.

Morley, D.A., Wilson, K. and McDermott, J. (2017) 'Changing the practice learning landscape', *Nurse Education in Practice*, 27, pp. 1–3.

Newton, J.M., Henderson, A., Jolly, B. and Greaves, J. (2014) 'A contemporary examination of workplace learning culture: An ethnomethodology study', *Nurse Education Today*, 35(1), pp. 91–99.

Nursing and Midwifery Council (NMC). (2018) Realising professionalism: Standards for education and training. Part 1: Standards framework for nursing and midwifery education. Available at: https://www.nmc.org.uk/globalassets/sitedocuments/education-standards/education-fram ework.pdf (accessed 03/14/19).

Pålsson, Y., Mårtensson, G., Swenne, C.L., Ädel, E. and Engström, M. (2017) 'A peer learning intervention for nursing students in clinical practice education: A quasi-experimental study', *Nurse Education Today*, 51, pp. 81–87.

Papastavrou, E., Lambrinou, E., Tsangari, H., Saarikoski, M. and Leino-Kilpi, H. (2010) 'Student nurses experience of learning in the clinical environment', *Nurse Education in Practice*, 10(3), pp. 176–182.

Papp, I., Markkanen, M. and von Bonsdorff, M. (2003) 'Clinical environment as a learning environment: student nurses' perceptions concerning clinical learning experiences', *Nurse Education Today*, 23(4), pp. 262–268.

Price, M., Rust, C., O'Donovan, B. Handley, K. and Bryant, R. (2012) *Assessment literacy: The foundation for improving student learning.* Oxford, UK: The Oxford Centre for Staff and Learning Development.

Race, P. (2014) *Making learning happen: A guide for post-compulsory education.* Third edition. London/ California/New Delhi/Singapore: Sage Publications Ltd.

Rohatinsky, N., Harding, K. and Carriere, T. (2017) 'Nursing student peer mentorship: A review of the literature', *Mentoring & Tutoring: Partnership in Learning*, 25(1), pp. 61–77.

Secomb, J. (2008) 'A systematic review of peer teaching and learning in clinical education', *Journal of Clinical Nursing*, 17(6), pp. 703–716.

Shipton, S.P. (2002) 'The process of seeking stress-care: Coping as experienced by senior baccalaureate nursing students in response to appraised clinical stress', *Journal of Nursing Education*, 41(6), pp. 243–256.

Smith, A., Beattie, M. and Kyle, R.G. (2015) 'Stepping up, stepping back, stepping forward: Student nurses' experiences as peer mentors in a pre-nursing scholarship', *Nurse Education in Practice*, 15(6), pp. 498–506.

Sprengel, A. D. and Job, L., (2004) 'Reducing student anxiety by using clinical peer mentoring with beginning nursing students', *Nurse Educator*, 29(6), pp. 245–250.

Walker, D., and Verklan, T. (2016) 'Peer mentoring during practicum to reduce anxiety in first-semester nursing students', *The Journal of Nursing Education*, 55(11), pp. 651–654.

Won, M. and Choi, Y. (2017) 'Undergraduate nursing student mentors' experiences of peer mentoring in Korea: A qualitative analysis', *Nurse Education Today*, 51, pp. 8–14.

4 Academic practice partnerships

Sinead Mehigan (s.mehigan@mdx.ac.uk), Laura Pisaneschi and Justin McDermott

Introduction

Nursing and midwifery are practice professions, and clinical practice learning must be central to their student education (Spence et al., 2012). The nursing profession needs to ensure that student nurses are provided with learning experiences in both academic and practice settings. If learners are to optimise practice learning to help them move beyond application of knowledge gained at university, to using their clinical reasoning skills in the practice setting, then collaborative working between academics and practitioners is essential. This means that academics and clinicians need to find ways of working in partnership so that all parties; learners, clinicians and academics are clear about roles, responsibilities, expectations and what needs to be enabled in practice and in higher education settings (Duffy et al., 2000; Bunce, 2002; Andrews et al., 2006).

There are wider benefits of such partnership working, in that quality education in the workplace is seen as key to driving improvements in patient care (Scott et al., 2017). The importance of establishing and sustaining learning cultures in clinical settings was highlighted in a report written by Francis (2013) as key to ensuring effective and compassionate nursing care. Close partnership working between academics and clinicians is essential to practice learning and especially if a student is struggling in practice (Skingley et al., 2007; Luhanga, Yonge and Myrick, 2008; Carlisle, Calman and Ibbotson, 2009). Yet partnership working can present huge challenges to both universities and clinical providers. Some of these challenges are logistical with, for example, busy academics and clinicians working in geographically diverse areas. Challenges can also arise when students themselves do not appreciate the importance of partnership working.

The purpose of this chapter is to critically reflect on the kinds of partnerships that help sustain effective clinical learning environments. This is timely, given the increasing emphasis on the importance of partnership working in the UK, with the NMC requiring greater transparency of how all partners work together to prepare learners for registration under new education standards (NMC, 2018b). These standards also require new professional roles, developed in partnership, to support learning and assessment in practice that potentially add complexity to the nature of partnership working. This chapter will highlight some of the factors and processes that influence partnership working for students in practice.

Many terms are used to define roles that support the learner in practice and these can sometimes be confusing. In this chapter we refer to the link lecturer (also known as link tutor) as an academic role and the practice educator (also known as clinical practice manager/facilitator, clinical practice educator) as a clinically based role.

Literature review

The literature refers to roles that exist to support learning in clinical practice in the UK, including that of the link lecturer. This is a potentially valuable role, where a nursing academic 'links' in with a designated clinical area, to support clinical staff and learners. However, the role has consistently been described as a difficult one to undertake. For example, link lecturers express uncertainty about their role in practice learning, particularly as they transition from practice to link lecturer, and how they maintain clinical credibility (Ramage, 2004). Tensions exist in maintaining links between clinical practice and education (Barrett, 2007; Carr, 2008; O'Driscoll, Allan and Smith, 2010).

Another support role within the UK is that of the lecturer-practitioner. Working in a joint capacity in both education and practice, Williamson (2004) suggests that this role has the potential to add value, particularly in bridging the theory-practice gap for learners. Other clinically based roles include that of a Practice Education Facilitator (PEF) (Carlisle et al., 2009; Sykes, Urquhart and Foster, 2014; Scott et al., 2017) or Clinical Practice Facilitator (Lambert and Glacken, 2006). Although all roles have been shown to be valuable, there seems to be recurring issues related to how they are defined, prepared for and supported.

Should university academics also work in the clinical setting?

Meskell, Murphy and Shaw (2009) suggest that the key to dynamic teaching in the classroom is remaining active in clinical practice. Pegram and Robinson (2002) indicate that one of the possible benefits of academics being actively involved in patient care is that it enhances classroom teaching although bringing critical incidents into the classroom to enhance teaching can raise issues of professional confidentiality. They advocate a third way of working between higher education and practice – that of adopting a model of faculty practice where lecturers gain honorary contracts to work with clinical providers in their areas of expertise for one day every two weeks. They draw on one model, designed to enable the lecturer as advanced practitioner to teach and as an educationalist to practice, and to facilitate research between the two areas. They found differing expectations of these roles, and issues were raised on academics' accountability for their continuity of decision making in practice.

The question of how realistic or sustainable it is to expect academics to remain clinically up to date is made by Carlisle et al. (2009), Sykes et al. (2014) and Scott et al. (2017). Workload demands for both academics and clinicians (Lambert and Glacken, 2006; Carnwell et al., 2007) create challenges for supporting learners in practice. Participants in Carnwell et al.'s (2007) study of link lecturers, lecturer-practitioners and mentors indicated that all experience role conflict by 'serving two masters'.

How can practice and academic staff work in partnership with learners?

Given the tensions already identified, other ways need to be found to build and sustain partnerships between universities and clinical practice.

From a student perspective, one of the key messages arising from the data (Andrews et al., 2006; Brown et al., 2005) was the importance they placed on having a member of the academic team visit them – whether because they felt alone in placement, wanted motivation to learn or recognised that they might take on a monitoring function. Although students realised that they had clinical staff to support their learning, there was recognition of the impact of workloads on clinicians' abilities to be able to support them. Students in Andrews et al.'s study (2006) indicated that the best models of placement support were where there were clear lines of communication and working between academics, mentors and clinical managers. However, although students recognised the formal routes highlighted in most clinical areas for contacting academics when in practice, they expressed reluctance to do so. This could infer something serious had occurred or that contacting their links might result in an assumption that the student was failing. These perceptions mirror anecdotal feedback the current authors have had from students.

One possibility to address students' concerns is the use of roles variously described as Practice Education Facilitators (PEFs) or Clinical Practice Facilitators (CPFs). These roles are diverse from supporting supervisory staff to conducting placement evaluations (Carlisle et al., 2009). Some of the benefits of these roles are that many have been set up specifically to help develop stronger links between universities and clinical practice settings (Carlisle et al., 2009; Sykes et al., 2014; Scott et al., 2017) and liaise between both settings in managing placement issues. The proximity to practice areas means that should issues arise, they are able to respond more readily than academics, in terms of supporting mentors and students (Carnwell et al., 2007; Scott et al., 2017). Their role is also seen to bridge theory and practice, given their familiarity with both university and clinical practice policies and processes (Scott et al., 2017).

Challenges to the role include a proliferation of role titles, with lack of clarity on the remit of the role, a lack of preparation (Coates and Fraser, 2014; Scott et al., 2017), and feelings of isolation and of being overwhelmed with the scope of the role (Lambert and Glacken, 2006). When these roles are too costly to support they can be vulnerable despite perceived benefits (Scott et al., 2017). O'Driscoll et al.'s study (2010) found uncertainty over roles, lack of support in practice for link lecturers, and workloads took precedence over supporting learners for clinical managers and mentors.

Within the US, there has been an increasing focus on the need for academics and clinicians to work together more effectively in partnership (Bakewell-Sachs, 2016). The Institute of Medicine (2010) proposed the adoption of a wider vision of academic nursing. This changing focus has culminated in a report from the American Association of Colleges of Nursing (2016) with recommendations to create an imperative for academic and clinical nurse leaders to work together with other healthcare leaders to 'realise the full benefits of academic nursing' (Sebastian et al., 2018, p. 110). Greater integration of nursing programmes with practice settings in Dedicated Education Units, as seen in examples from Australia and the USA, find clinicians and academics working together in practice, research and the implementation of educational programmes (Edgecombe et al., 1999; Moscato et al., 2007; Ranse and Grealish, 2007).

Carnwell et al. (2007) offer an alternative option, that of a team approach to mentoring, along the lines of an Australian model. There, learners are placed in practice areas two days each week for a whole semester, and mentors ensure that students gain access to relevant learning opportunities. Lecturer practitioners are involved in teaching specific skills, in assessing and supervising. This seems to resonate with the NMC (2018b) standards for supporting learners in practice. Spence et al. (2012) adopted and evaluated a 'student integration model' in New Zealand, similar to the one currently used in the UK, where learners were considered part of the team, working with a range of healthcare workers under the supervision of a registered nurse who acted as a mentor. Different models of mentoring and coaching related to a team-based approach to learning are further discussed in Chapter 5, 'Expansive learning'.

Methodology

A mixed methods approach was used to gather data from stakeholders. Qualitative analysis from feedback from two group meetings was used – one was a large event, made up of clinical educators, and the other a smaller meeting of academics and clinicians. Qualitative analysis was employed using first level coding as a retrieval device to facilitate identification of recurring themes (Miles and Huberman, 1994). Inter-reliability for thematic analysis was used by two researchers to summarise key findings from both sets of data. The first set of data collected came from focus group one, a 2017 London Association of Mental Health Nursing Practice (LAMP) conference where 179 participants were asked to respond in groups to three questions. The group consisted of practitioners (the majority working in the field of mental health) representing hospitals and universities across the whole London region. A summary of discussions on each table was captured by a facilitator on a flip chart. The questions posed were:

1   What aspects of the role of the link lecturer do you most value?
2   What support / resources do you feel could enhance your role in supporting student learning and assessment in practice?
3   Are there examples of resources / activities you use or are available to you now that work well?

The second set of data came from focus group two with 15 participants comprising of recently registered nurses and nurse academics. The group were asked to consider three questions on the topic of Academic and Practice Partnerships. The key points raised from discussions were captured by a facilitator on each table using an on-line data capture app called Padlet. The questions used to generate discussion were:

In relation to partnership working between HEI's, employers, stakeholders:

1   What works?
2   What does not work?
3   What needs to change?

Results

Six themes emerged from the findings:

1. Preparation

The issue of preparation was raised in both focus groups for academics and clinicians, for roles in supporting learning and assessment in practice. For clinicians, "Prior warning – allocating students" (focus group 2) and to receive regular information about changes in nursing education "Training updates e.g. recent changes in PAD [Practice Assessment Document]" was important (focus group 2). For clinicians being prepared meant having timely information about when students were coming and updates on student assessment and mentor updates, "Mentors to be informed well in advance when students are coming to clinical placements to enable them to prepare and welcome them" (focus group 2).

Academics in the second focus group felt there was an assumption that they knew what to do but that this did not reflect their reality especially regarding the transition from clinician to link lecturer, which had been more difficult than they had anticipated. The second focus group stated the importance of being prepared to succeed as a link lecturer, "Preparation is key" (focus group 2).

"Protected time with students/time to complete paperwork" (focus group 1) and "protected time (coaching, reflecting, teaching, time with students)" (focus group 1) was highlighted.

2. Roles

Focus groups discussed the role of the link lecturer and their role in providing support and guidance for mentors. They requested for "roles and responsibilities being clarified" (focus group 1), "agreeing mutual goals – and ensure these are known at all levels of the organisation" (focus group 2) and identified the "need to work together within and between organisations to make things clearer – peer support for learners can help increase clarity of roles and support" (focus group 2).

3. Accessibility

Much of the feedback, particularly from participants in focus group one suggested the importance of link lecturers being present with "regular visits and feedback" (focus group 1) with "link lecturers to have a set time for contact so students expect when they come in" (focus group 1). Many of the comments repeated the importance of clinicians knowing how to contact link lecturers if needed.

For some, it was important for partnership working that clinicians were engaged with the higher education institution (HEI). This engagement entailed the development and communication of policies, processes, procedure and/or the overall governance/management of student education. Being engaged in education updates and curriculum development meant that clinicians led in the discussion of practice learning and how this relates to frameworks for learning across all areas; "arranging to meet with clinicians, actively engaging them in updates". Academics also provided a route to current evidence-based practice "bridging the gap between theory and practice" (focus group 2). Both focus groups highlighted the importance of academic staff being present both at assessment and in the development of resources, and the potential for the "opportunity for mentors to spend time in the university" (focus group 1).

The need for protected time to undertake more effective learning and assessment was highlighted throughout, particularly for clinicians undertaking mentor or education support roles. Several participants stated they valued the role of the PEF which in some areas has replaced the link lecturer. PEFs were seen to have a valuable support role for mentors in practice, not least because of their proximity and ability to be more accessible if problems arose. PEF's have, in these areas, increasingly taken over the role of the link lecturer in terms of supporting mentors, clinical teams and students in practice – often as a result of time pressures on link lecturers due to conflicting academic workloads.

4. Networking

Participants in both focus groups highlighted the need for more support for those staff that are responsible for learning and assessment in practice. From the clinician's perspective, support was not only needed from academics and the HEI, but also "support from managers so student and mentor work together" (focus group 1). "Shared learning experience across clinical disciplines and areas" (focus group 1) such as "attendance at LAMP conferences" (focus group 1) were identified. Data indicated the need for a "partnership approach within an organisation, to facilitate student focused sessions" (focus group 2) through shared negotiation in terms of planning, reviewing goals and working together for a common aim. Participants recognised the value of partnership in teaching and decision making and the need to ensure a consistent approach.

5. Communication

Both focus groups highlighted that "communication is key" (focus group 2). "Being available and responsive" (focus group 2) was important to building regular communication particularly with the link lecturer. Participants emphasised the importance of building a relationship, communication between all parties and of maintaining a good rapport so "both parties collaborate" (focus group 2) especially in the light of poor communications when "relationships between universities and placements communication can fail and not work" (focus group 2). The importance of face to face communication as well as the use of email and telephone was identified and strengthened through inductions and partnership working.

6. Expertise

Some mentors thought that the link lecturer should be the person bringing their expertise and up to date knowledge to the practice setting. They were "resourceful" and "we value their existence" (focus group 1). However, in focus group two there was more emphasis on knowledge exchange between the clinicians (mentors) and academic staff. Sharing learning opportunities was identified, "good to have clinicians and academics working together" (focus group 2), with the opportunity of inviting clinicians into the university to teach. The data showed that there are some excellent resources and learning activities already established in partnership areas such as "learning resource packs for both students and nurses" (focus group 1) and conferences.

The six themes from the results can be categorised into a model which is useful in both theory and practice. The model encompassing the six themes is PRANCE which is made up of: Preparation, Responsibilities, Accessibility, Networking, Communication and Expertise.

Analysis

The findings demonstrate that there is a real sense that staff working in practice with learners do need support from their own organisations in terms of being allocated time and recognition from their managers or having additional support roles, such as PEFs (Carlisle et al., 2009; Sykes et al., 2014; Scott et al., 2017). Participants also value and need close working with link lecturers from HEIs. Academics are seen to bring expertise about the programme content, the students themselves and how to negotiate difficult or challenging issues related to teaching and assessment in practice. They are also seen, to a lesser extent, as another resource in terms of giving access to wider research findings. Key to providing support is the need to be accessible and present – however, participants in our study reflected wider research in recognising that HEI commitments meant that link lecturers could not always be present when needed and that their current dual workloads were challenging (Lambert and Glacken, 2006; Carnwell et al., 2007).

There is recognition, from both academics and clinicians, of the need within the existing system of student support for good preparation for both sets of staff. Some of this relates to having clear role expectations and knowing that timely guidance, information and updates on student progression will be available. This links with findings from other studies, indicating issues such as uncertainty over roles and lack of support or workloads impacts on the quality of student support given (O'Driscoll et al., 2010). Given that the current systems of student support have been in place for some time, with a re-framing of how student support and assessment need to be undertaken (NMC, 2018b), there is an opportunity to revise and update current approaches – particularly in situations where one clinical area might expect to support students from a number of different higher education institutions.

Feedback from clinicians and academics in our study shows that they recognise the importance of working together to support students in practice. There is evidence of a range of strategies and resources that have been developed to help with this process, including preparation of clinical staff to take on student support roles, and ongoing communication and direct support to assist with student assessment. Much of the support highlighted in the study reflects current NMC requirements for supporting and assessing learners in practice.

Conclusion

Academic-practice partnership working is beneficial to preparing future generations of students to gain professional registration and to ensure continuing excellence in healthcare provision by promoting consistency between education at university and education in practice.

Findings from the literature, and from data collected for this chapter, present clear messages of what is needed to ensure effective clinical learning environments for nursing students. What did not emerge from the data was Meskell et al.'s (2009) notion that key to dynamic teaching in the classroom was clinical immersion in clinical practice. The focus from data was on what clinicians and academics needed to do to support learning in practice. Staff across academic and clinical areas finding ways of working together to define what is needed and develop clear role definitions are important so that expectations and standards are aligned across practice and academic areas with no gulf between. At the micro level of student learning, Chapters 2 and 3 also highlight the potential role of unregistered health care staff and peer students to support student learning in partnership as 'helpful others'.

Staff and student participants identified the essential nature of preparation for their partnership roles. Although current practice supports preparation for mentorship, in the form of national professional body standards from the NMC (2018a), there seemed to be less consistency in the preparation of academics to support clinical learning in practice. This is something that is worth exploring further in future research and to seek the opinion of current students who were missing as participants in this study. With new standards for supporting partnership working, particularly in learning and assessment in practice (NMC, 2018a), there is an opportunity for organisations to re-examine how they work together in preparing and planning for clinicians and academics to support students in practice. As the current standards are written, there is an emphasis for both the academic and clinician on taking a role as an assessor in the clinical setting as either a practice or an academic assessor. The challenge will be as to how organisations develop such roles so that the supportive elements of partnership are not lost.

The study findings found a lack of clarity around current roles to support learners in practice although clear definitions and developmental pathways for their development have existed for some time, as outlined in the SLAiP standards (NMC, 2008). There is a need for organisations to commit to working closely together to develop shared approaches in the preparation and ongoing development of academic and practice staff so that there is clarity of the new partnership roles of practice supervisor and practice assessor. The interpretation of these roles may differ and reflect local aspects such as staffing, services or capacity. The challenges assessors and supervisors face with the NMC standards (2018) is one of ensuring that the principles of assessment (reliability, validity, robustness) are communicated effectively. The onus is on practice assessors/supervisors to articulate what the learner knows, needs to know, how they are to do this and whether they have achieved set learning outcomes. This needs to be enacted with the learner at the centre and their development facilitated in line with the proficiencies and professional values required for the respective level.

Existing studies, and this study, suggests that internal and external conflicts, competing demands and requirements and a lack of clear, timely and open channels of communications can all contribute to a breakdown in partnership working. The emergence of new routes into nursing, such as apprenticeships, will require additional partnership working as the practice learning setting negotiates a greater diversity of learner roles. In reviewing what is required for effective partnership working, the adoption of the steps identified previously as PRANCE (Preparation, Responsibilities, Accessibility, Networking, Communication and Expertise) are recommended.

Recommendations

Our recommendations for academic-practice partnership focus on the key areas from PRANCE (Preparation, Roles, Accessibility, Networking, Communication, Expertise):

Preparation

Clear processes for the preparation of each role in partnership learning, and provision of a forum to enable sharing of expertise and experiences are seen as fundamental. Preparation could take the form of sufficient training and updates as well as joint Practice Education Teams and meetings.

Responsibility

Clarity on responsibilities and any respective accountability will ensure the student receives a positive and connected experience between their academic and practice learning. Role descriptors, and a clearly defined process that is transparent to all, would be beneficial and result in the most efficient use of resource.

Accessibility

The identification of how education institutions and practice areas support partnership needs to be accurately identified. This could be how, when, who can be contacted and what support is available should the contact person not be available. Consideration should be given to response times in urgent and priority circumstances.

Networking

A team-based, collaborative approach to academic-practice partnership is recommended with clear guidance on the practical workings of the partnership to enable each to expand on their knowledge and understanding of the practice learning environment and learners. Being able to contact others in an organisation easily, and in pre agreed meetings, could result in the recognition of further learning opportunities and the enhancement of learners' skills.

Communication

The foundation of academic-practice partnerships is effective communication and this will be particularly important with the implementation of the new professional roles for assessment. We would recommend a mixed economy of online means of communication, such as webinars, due to geographical distances but also prearranged face to face meetings to encourage more personalised discourse. Various means of communication can be explored (i.e. in person, virtual) with the emphasis on the quality of the exchanges. Resources should be created to direct and signpost those involved.

Expertise

We recommend that each person in the partnership will have their respective knowledge and can bring this expertise in ensuring the learning is supported and enhanced. The recognition of this, be it clinical or academic skills and knowledge, will help all those involved in the partnership of enhancing learning. The data from the two focus groups showed that there are some excellent resources and learning activities established already in partnership areas such as learning packs and conferences.

Case Study for Academic Practice Partnerships

This case study uses the steps identified as PRANCE (Preparation, Roles, Accessibility, Networking, Communication, Expertise) to highlight how key aspects of partnership working can be met in supporting learning and assessment in practice. These steps can be considered in any order and the mnemonic is provided as a resource to aid recall when required.

The student scenario used in this case study considers of the roles of Practice Supervisors (PS), Practice Assessor (PA) and Academic Assessor as required within the Standards for Student Supervision and Assessment (NMC, 2018b).

Joseph is a Year 2 student nurse starting his final placement of the year in a community setting. Previous placements in Year 2 have been within a hospital and so this is a completely new practice area where he is very anxious about achieving the required outcomes.

What is the learning aim?

To establish an effective partnership approach to facilitate a positive learning experience, achievement of proficiencies and support progression to the next part of the education programme for Joseph.

What learning will be achieved?

1   To ensure adequate preparation for practice to enable Joseph to take a proactive role in directing his own learning.
2   To facilitate appropriate learning opportunities for Joseph and ensure a consistent approach to supervision and support.
3   To facilitate a partnership approach to Joseph's assessment of practice.

How can learning be supported?

1 To ensure adequate preparation for practice to enable Joseph to take a proactive role in directing his own learning

Preparation by the university, which is further enhanced in the practice area, can support socialisation and promote a positive learning culture (Bakewell-Sachs, 2016). Ensuring Joseph understands the potential learning opportunities, and how these relate to his objectives and assessment requirements, will empower him and enable him to be a key partner in this learning relationship. A clear understanding of the **R**oles of the Practice Supervisor, Practice Assessor and Academic Assessor, and how to contact them, will support a successful experience.

2 To facilitate a range of appropriate learning opportunities for Joseph and ensure a consistent approach to supervision and support

Accessibility is an important concept in the student learning experience so Joseph can contact a nominated person with whom he can raise concerns and also be supported by all staff appropriate to his learning in the practice setting. Expanding Joseph's learning opportunities beyond the local team (**N**etworking) may inspire him, enhance his learning and promote a sense of feeling valued (HEE, 2018). Access to a range of appropriately prepared registered health and social care professionals who can supervise learning and contribute to assessment will aid his learning (NMC, 2018b) when they work in a coordinated network to provide Joseph with a variety of relevant practice learning experiences.

3 To facilitate a partnership approach to Joseph's assessment of practice

Communication between the partnership members and most particularly with the Practice Supervisor and Academic Assessor is key. Clarity of roles will ensure partnerships are not blurred to the extent gaps appear and Joseph has elements of his practice either not recognised or misinterpreted. This will also support the networking between supervisors and assessors so that each person in Joseph's education is represented. Each person in the partnership, including Joseph, will bring their respective knowledge and **E**xpertise to this relationship and all have important roles in creating a positive experience.

References

American Association of Colleges of Nursing. (2016) Advancing health care transformation: A new era for academic nursing. Washington, DC: Author. Available at: www.aacn.nche.edu/AACN-Manatt-Report.pdf.

Andrews, G., Brodie, D., Andrews, J., Hillan, E., Gail Thomas, B., Wong, J. and Rixon, L. (2006) 'Professional roles and communications in clinical placements: A qualitative study of nursing students' perceptions and some models for practice', *International Journal of Nursing Studies*, 43(7), pp. 861–874.

Bakewell-Sachs, S. (2016) 'Academic-practice partnerships driving and supporting educational changes', *Journal of Perinatal & Neonatal Nursing*, 30(3), pp. 184–186.

Barrett, D. (2007) 'The clinical role of nurse lecturers: Past, present, and future', *Nurse Education Today*, 27(5), pp. 367–374.

Breslin, E., Sebastian, J., Trautman, D., Cary, A., Rosseter, R. and Vlahov, D. (2018) 'Leadership by collaboration: Nursing's bold new vision for academic-practice partnerships', *Journal of Professional Nursing*, 34(1), pp. 110–116.

Brown, L., Herd, K., Humphries, G. and Paton, M. (2005) 'The role of the lecturer in practice placements: What do students think?' *Nurse Education in Practice*, 5(2), pp. 84–90.

Bunce, C. (2002) 'Placement blues', *Nursing Times*, 98(17), pp. 24–26.

Carlisle, C., Calman, L. and Ibbotson, T. (2009) 'Practice-based learning: The role of practice education facilitators in supporting mentors', *Nurse Education Today*, 29(7), pp. 715–721.

Carnwell, R., Baker, S., Bellis, M. and Murray, R. (2007) 'Managerial perceptions of mentor, lecturer practitioner and link tutor roles', *Nurse Education Today*, 27(8), pp. 923–932.

Carr, J. (2008) 'Mentoring student nurses in the practice', *Practice Nursing*, 19(9), pp. 465–467.

Coates, K. and Fraser, K. (2014) 'A case for collaborative networks for clinical nurse educators', *Nurse Education Today*, 34(1), pp. 6–10.

Duffy, K., Docherty, C., Cardnuff, L., White, M., Winters, G. and Greig, J. (2000) 'The nurse lecturer's role in mentoring the mentors', *Nursing Standard*, 15(6), pp. 35–38.

Edgecombe, K., Wotton, K., Gonda, J. and Mason, P. (1999) 'Dedicated education units: 1 A new concept for clinical teaching and learning', *Contemporary Nurse*, 8(4), pp. 166–171.

Francis, R. (2013) *Mid Staffordshire NHS Foundation Trust public inquiry*. London: The Stationary Office. Available at: http://tinyurl.com/p2ebw82 (accessed 07/30/18).

Health Education England (HEE). (2018) RePAIR: Reducing pre-registration attrition and improving retention report. Available at: https://www.hee.nhs.uk/our-work/reducing-pre-re gistration-attrition-improving-retention (accessed 02/11/18).

Institute of Medicine. (2010) *The future of nursing: Leading change, advancing health*. Washington, DC: The National Academies Press.

Lambert, V. and Glacken, M. (2006) 'Clinical education facilitators' and post-registration paediatric student nurses' perceptions of the role of the clinical education facilitator', *Nurse Education Today*, 26(5), pp. 358–366.

Luhanga, F., Yonge, O. and Myrick, F. (2008) 'Precepting an unsafe student: The role of the faculty', *Nurse Education Today*, 28(2), pp. 227–231.

Meskell, P., Murphy, K. and Shaw, D. (2009) 'The clinical role of lecturers in nursing in Ireland: Perceptions from key stakeholder groups in nurse education on the role', *Nurse Education Today*, 29(7), pp. 784–790.

Miles, M. and Huberman, A. (1994) *Qualitative data analysis: A methods sourcebook*, 3. London: Sage Publications, Inc.

Moscato, S., Miller, J., Logsdon, K., Weinberg, S. and Chorpenning, L. (2007) 'Dedicated education unit: An innovative clinical partner education model', *Nursing Outlook*, 55(1), pp. 31–37.

Nursing and Midwifery Council (NMC). (2008) *Standards to support learning and assessment in practice*. Available at: https://www.nmc.org.uk/globalassets/sitedocuments/standards/nmc-standa rds-to-support-learning-assessment.pdf (accessed 11/16/18).

Nursing and Midwifery Council (NMC). (2018) 'Standards for nurses'. Available at: https://www. nmc.org.uk/standards/standards-for-nurses/ (accessed 06/11/18).

Nursing and Midwifery Council (NMC). (2018a) 'Part 1: Standards for nursing and midwifery education'. Available at: https://www.nmc.org.uk/globalassets/sitedocuments/education-standa rds/education-framework.pdf (accessed 05/21/18).

Nursing and Midwifery Council (NMC). (2018b) 'Part 2: Standards for student supervision and assessment'. Available at: https://www.nmc.org.uk/standards-for-education-and-training/standa rds-for-student-supervision-and-assessment/ (accessed 06/18).

O'Driscoll, M.F., Allan, H.T. and Smith, P.A. (2010) 'Still looking for leadership – Who is responsible for student nurses' learning in practice?' *Nurse Education Today*, 30(3), pp. 212–217.

Pegram, A. and Robinson, L. (2002) 'The experience of undertaking faculty practice', *Nurse Education in Practice*, 2(1), pp. 30–34.

Ramage, C. (2004) 'Negotiating multiple roles: Link teachers in clinical nursing practice', *Journal of Advanced Nursing*, 45(3), pp. 287–296.

Ranse, K. and Grealish, L. (2007) 'Nursing students' perceptions of learning in the clinical setting of the Dedicated Education Unit', *Journal of Advanced Nursing*, 58(2), pp. 171–179.

Scott, B., Rapson, T., Allibone, L., Hamilton, R., Mambanje, C. and Pisaneschi, L. (2017) 'Practice education facilitator roles and their value to NHS organisations', *British Journal of Nursing*, 26 (4), pp. 222–227.

Sebastian, J.G., Breslin, E.T., Trautman, D.E., Cary, A.H., Rosseter, R.J. and Vlahov, D. (2018) 'Leadership by collaboration: Nursing's bold new vision for academic-practice partnerships', *Journal of Professional Nursing*, 34(2), pp. 110–116.

Skingley, A., Arnott, J., Greaves, J. and Nabb, J. (2007) 'Supporting practice teachers to identify failing students', *British Journal of Community Nursing*, 12(1), pp. 28–32.

Spence, D., Valiant, S., Roud, D. and Aspinall, C. (2012) 'Preparing registered nurses depends on "us and us and all of us"', *Nursing praxis in New Zealand inc*, 28(2), pp. 5.

Sykes, C., Urquhart, C. and Foster, A. (2014) 'Role of the Practice Education Facilitator (PEF): The Cambridgeshire model underpinned by a literature review of educational facilitator roles', *Nurse Education Today*, 34(11), pp. 1395–1397.

Williamson, G.R. (2004) 'Lecturer practitioners in UK nursing and midwifery: What is the evidence? A systematic review of the research literature', *Journal of Clinical Nursing*, 13(7), pp. 787–795.

5 Expansive learning

Natalie Holbery (natholbery@gmail.com), Dawn A. Morley and Joady Mitchell

Introduction

Chapter 5 explores the concept of 'expansive learning' taken from Fuller and Unwin's (2003) research of apprenticeships where they identified a 'restrictive–expansive continuum' that classified the type of learning environment presented in the work place. Crucially, expansive learning encouraged a supportive environment for students to learn higher level skills such as dialogue, problem solving and reflexive forms of expertise.

Supportive and collaborative learning environments can instil confidence in the student to develop and the practice supervisory role (or previously the mentor) is significant to this. The chapter theme of expansive learning is led by the goal to discover what teaching and learning processes can assist all levels of clinical staff in supporting students to move effectively, and in a well-supported way, to the expertise or 'graduateness' (Eden, 2014) required at registration and beyond. This was an important foundation of the recent NMC (2017) review.

Chapter 2 and Chapter 3 have already demonstrated the potential educational role of unregistered staff and peer students who previously have not been officially recognised for coaching learners in practice. With focused and explicit support for their learning, students' placement experience can be 'supercharged' so their learning advances quicker and with greater impact on their long term professional development (Morley, 2018).

A model of coaching that emerged from the research study is also presented. Current emphasis in practice learning is placed on the assessment of measurable clinical skills rather than the students' ability to join these skills holistically in professional practice (Morley, 2015). The ability to be able to teach this type of integration of student performance into the busy clinical practice is more akin to the fluidity of 'coaching' rather than 'teaching' and this is explored fully within the chapter.

Literature review

Ellstrom (2011) made the distinction between an enabling and constraining learning environment whereby the structures in the practice setting impact on how easily a student can move between adaptive (skills acquisition) and developmental (professional critique) learning. A constraining working environment could prioritise adaptive learning, or be detrimental to the development of both, with students displaying acquiescence. Although the prioritisation of adaptive or developmental learning may naturally and appropriately occur during their learning, students need encouragement to be able to question what and how they are being taught in order to achieve graduate skills.

Are students able to achieve their learning potential in practice through expansive learning?

Benner's (1984) insights into the possibility of making nurses' practice learning more proactive have been influential to the debate on how practice learning is taught. Significantly, Benner (1984) believed that the skilled pattern recognition of experts could be taught, rather than being incidental, and the learning emphasis should be placed on the whole of practice and not the isolation of component skills. Morley (2018) found that if students' supervision was handed over to unregistered staff, such as health care assistants, students developed a fragmented view of care with a division between essential nursing care and the management of the clinical area. Only by working with their formal supervisor (previously called a mentor) could nurses develop the 360-degree awareness of both the management and the care together. By observing the work of an expert in action, student nurses enjoyed the rare opportunity for a more holistic view on practice learning where their learning was brought together in one event (Spouse, 2001; Morley, 2018). Benner (1984) believed that one of the essential differences between a novice and expert nurse is that the former will view clinical incidents as a compilation of different parts rather than a whole. The join up of all the disparate parts of practice learning could be embodied in the practice of the expert but significantly this could not be learnt if students did not have consistent quality time with their supervisor.

The type of supervision experienced by students could therefore delay their progression to graduate type skills (Gray and Smith, 1999; Mackintosh, 2006). Traditionally, the lack of support of student nurses has led to cases of bullying and an inability of the student to find their own voice and be an advocate for their clients (Morley, 2018).

Why is it important for student nurses to be able to think and action a more critical, expansive learning approach to their practice?

Schon (1983) argued that the complexity of professional decision making needed to accommodate for the unplanned circumstances of practice. If students were socialised to reacting in frequently occurring clinical situations, then students would fail to manage the many unplanned circumstances of practice. Strengthening student attributes of self-regulation (Kuiper and Pesut, 2004) and emotional resilience (Grant and Kinman, 2014) are synonymous with the promotion of expansive learning and the identified professional need for registered nurses and midwives to be advocates for their patients (NMC, 2017) as well as being able to support a professional duty of candour about their practice (NMC, 2018).

Brown and Duguid (1991) found that organisational structures meant to assist practice could also form barriers to practice and learning. There is the risk, for example, that the present documentation of assessment in practice learning could constrain student nurses' practice learning in missing the more implicit aspects of learning in practice. The documentation emphasises the achievement of individually achieved practice skills rather than the whole of practice through collaborative working.

The literature suggests that a more fluid model of learning may be appropriate to the practice setting rather than one that is restricted by the measurement of competency alone (Morley, 2015).

What learning strategies help promote expansive learning?

Although immersion into practice can give students the opportunity to observe and imitate the complexities of professional practice (the tacit dimension) (Harteis et al., 2012), the busyness of practice can also obscure the learning that students have undertaken (Morley, 2015). Benner (1984) and Eraut (2000, 2004) highlighted the risks of learning not being made explicit enough for students to recognise.

Argyris and Schon (1974) described the mechanism of resolving practice issues within the given variables of a setting as 'single loop learning'. By reflecting on problems innovatively the gulf between theory and practice is bridged by what Argyris and Schon (1974) described as 'double loop learning' where the work setting is critically scrutinised for more innovative solutions. Argyris and Schon's work therefore highlights whether appropriate pedagogy, such as reflection, could enable students to more easily challenge accepted practice.

Schon's (1983) reflection in action provides a possible mechanism for student nurses to elicit learning from their practice whereby a professional incorporates intended real-time reflection into their practice. Although criticised for the separation of the act of reflection from action, Schon introduced coaching, rather than teaching mechanisms that explicitly built on previous knowledge and the development of a critical appreciation of practice (Gobbi, 2012).

What coaching models promote expansive learning?

Coaching has become a recognised part of student development across all disciplines where students are taught peer coaching strategies (Burns and Gillon, 2011) or have named individuals (Eccles and Renaud, 2018) guiding them at particular points, such as placements, during their programmes.

Changes to the clinical student support structure for student nurses and midwives (NMC, 2018) recognised the potential difficulties, and compromise, that the former mentor role took when combining the coaching and assessing of students. There has been growing interest in alternative coaching approaches for students in practice (Bazian, 2016); most notably the CLiP (Collaborative Learning in Practice) model, highlighted by Willis's second enquiry (2015).

The principles of the CLiP model lie in the development of 'real world' clinical areas where up to 20 students deliver care, identify their own learning outcomes and are more explicitly coached in small groups by a member of registered staff. This role is their sole responsibility during the shift. In their turn, a clinical educator oversees a wider clinical area and guides the coaches (Lobo, Arthur and Lattimer, 2014; Huggins, 2016; HEE, 2017). Huggins (2016) and HEE (2017) show early indications of increased student, supervisor and patient satisfaction, with students articulating increased knowledge and confidence due to the considerable investment made in coaching. On evaluation, student opinion was divided as to whether they lacked opportunity and autonomy or whether they had had a greater opportunity to work as a staff nurse (Hill, Woodward and Arthur, 2015).

The success of CLiP is dependent on close, collaborative working and a shared ethos across practice partners, 'positive ward culture was the most significant feature for successful CLiP implementation; a culture receptive to change and educationally focused . . . as was strong and positive leadership' (Hill et al., 2015, p. 1). The coach receiving support and additional training from a clinical educator proved crucial and, like the mentor before them, 'staffing levels within the placement area were considered to be the most important factor in ensuring that the role of the coach was effective' (p. 1). Without adequate staffing levels there was a risk that clinical educators became replacement coaches themselves and students reverted to peer teaching as the only form of support and guidance. Where there was a difference in the experience of students in a peer mentoring relationship then coaching was beneficial but held 'the potential to mask poorly supervised student practice' if not (Hill et al., 2015, p. 23). It was also found that staff in other areas of the ward were reluctant to enter CLiP teaching bays and this also restricted the learning of students to elsewhere in the clinical area (Hill et al., 2015).

The scarcity of published evaluation remains a requirement on the CLiP model (Clarke, Williamson and Kane, 2018), and more research is needed on the suitability of the model across different settings and types of students. The model's applicability for senior students, for example, is an important area to investigate where students' liaison with the nurse in charge and other staff, such as health care assistants, is critical to their development as clinical managers (Morley, 2018).

Methodology

A six-month study was conducted in 2016–2017 and recruited 308 nursing and midwifery students representing various stages of their programme and from every field of nursing (adult, child and mental health). A total of 72 mentors from adult, child and mental health fields took part in separate focus groups.

Ethical approval was granted from the University's Ethics Committee.

Data collection methods

A short questionnaire was designed for student participants to elicit their views on 'good' mentoring and support whilst on placement. The questionnaire required one-word responses only. The researchers believed this approach would encourage students to reflect and consider their responses with care. The questionnaire was either completed in paper format at a student event (March 2017) or electronically (April 2017). Not all students completed all questions, hence the disparity in the number of responses noted.

1   Who has been most helpful with your learning on this placement?
2   What has this person done to best support your learning?
3   What is the most important thing you have learned from this person?
4   Which word best describes the attributes of a good mentor?
5   Which word best describes a good learning environment?

Twelve focus groups were conducted at three different events during January– April 2017 to elicit mentor views and understand their experience of one-to-one coaching (as opposed to mentoring) skills that help students achieve expansive learning. Mentors were briefed on the term 'expansive learning' and asked to conduct three activities as outlined in Table 5.1.

Table 5.1 Mentor focus group activities.

Activity	Data collection method
Individually record 5 coaching skills important to students in a 1:1 practice learning situation	Post-it Notes
In the focus group collate and review responses. Agree and merge duplicated skills.	Post-it Notes
In the focus group prioritise the coaching skills most useful for struggling and then excelling students	Flip chart & Post-it Notes

Data analysis methods

The student questionnaire responses were collated. Similar and plural words were merged and the most frequently occurring were represented using word cloud software, Wordle. Word clouds are a visual representation that display words according to the number of responses. Thematic analysis of data from the mentor focus groups was completed by three researchers. The phases of data analysis are outlined in Table 5.2.

Table 5.2 Phases of data analysis.

Phase 1	Identification of overarching themes
Phase 2	Exploration of themes relevant to coaching skills
Phase 3	Identification of the stages of a coaching model

Results and analysis

a From student questionnaires

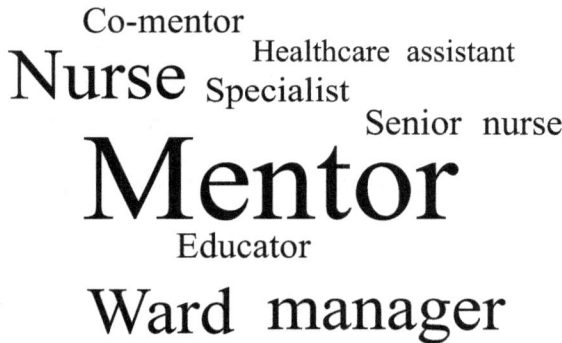

Figure 5.1 Who has been most helpful with your learning on this placement?

Table 5.3 Responses to 'Who has been most helpful with your learning on this placement?'

Result	Responses (n=242)	Result	Responses (n=242)
Mentor	96	Senior nurse/specialist	13
Nurse	47	Educator	11
Ward manager	37	Health care assistant	4
Co-mentor	12	Other	37

Student responses indicated a broad view on whom they saw as helpful to their learning. The term co-mentor, identified by students, refers to a nurse who supports learning in practice (in addition to a registered named mentor) but who does not have a formal mentorship qualification. This approach is commonly used in student placements to build mentorship capacity and/or support nurses during completion of a mentorship programme. Despite the potential duplication of identifying the same individuals in practice, for example, nurse and mentor, students tended to prioritise registered staff. However, 17 per cent of participants did identify individuals who may not have an officially recognised teaching role (health care assistant and other) identified as 'helpful others' in Chapter 2.

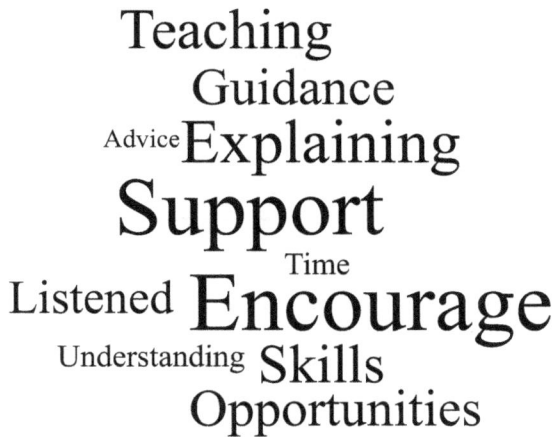

Figure 5.2 What has this person done to best support your learning?

Table 5.4 Responses to 'What has this person done to best support your learning?'

Result	Responses (n=241)	Result	Responses (n=241)
Support	29	Skills	14
Encourage	27	Listened	13
Explaining	19	Understanding	7
Guidance	15	Time	7
Teaching	15	Advice	4
Opportunities	15	Others	83

The student participants placed great value on interpersonal skills as important to supporting their learning in practice. Many of these words represent a facilitative, rather than didactic, approach which also reflects the themes drawn out from the mentor focus groups and is aligned to findings from other studies (Chapman, 2001; D'Souza et al., 2015; Sundler et al., 2014). Whilst this focus, on developing interpersonal skills, is lacking in current mentorship education, McIntosh, Gidman and Smith (2013) found that mentors are aware that their personal attributes were important to successfully supporting learning in practice.

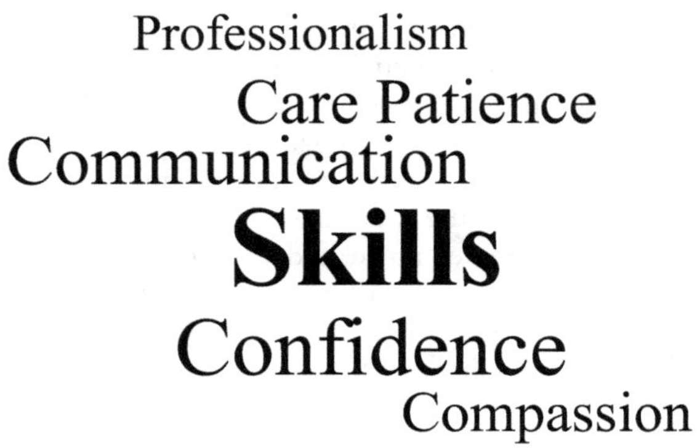

Professionalism
Care Patience
Communication

Skills

Confidence
Compassion

Figure 5.3 What is the most important thing you have learned from this person?

Table 5.5 Responses to 'What is the most important thing you have learned from this person?'

Result	Responses (n=234)	Result	Responses (n=234)
Skills	26	Patience	10
Confidence	15	Compassion	9
Communication	12	Professionalism	8
Care	11	Other	185

The results were limited by the lack of specific definition, but participants identified that their practice learning has been an amalgamation of all types of professional learning from practical skills to attributes such as compassion.

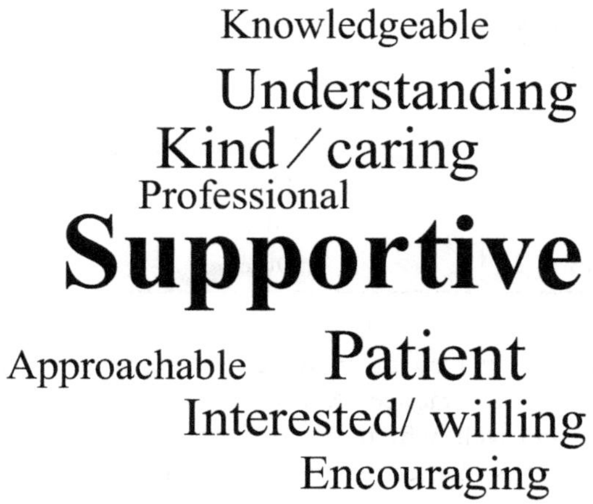

Knowledgeable

Understanding
Kind / caring
Professional

Supportive

Approachable   Patient
Interested/ willing
Encouraging

Figure 5.4 Which word best describes the attributes of a good mentor?

Table 5.6 Responses to 'What is the most important thing you have learned from this person?'

Result	Responses (n=240)	Result	Responses (n=240)
Supportive	44	Encouraging	10
Patient	24	Knowledgeable	8
Kind/caring	16	Approachable	8
Understanding	15	Professional	7
Interested/willing	12	Others	96

Interpersonal skills were the key features identified as important mentor attributes although 40 per cent of responses were classified as 'others'. The largest term identified at 18 per cent was being supportive.

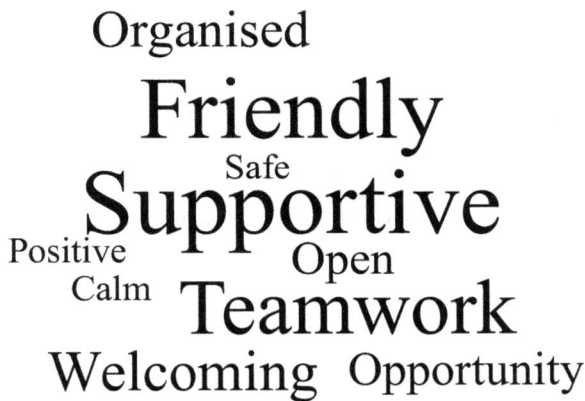

Organised

Friendly

Safe

Supportive

Positive   Open

Calm   Teamwork

Welcoming   Opportunity

Figure 5.5 Which word best describes a good learning environment?

Table 5.7 Responses to 'Which word best describes a good learning environment?'

Result	Responses (n=234)	Result	Responses (n=234)
Supportive	26	Open	8
Friendly	23	Calm	7
Teamwork	19	Positive	7
Welcoming	14	Safe	6
Organised	12	Other	102
Opportunity	10		

Interpersonal factors, and particularly that of being supportive and friendly, feature as important for a good learning environment. It is interesting to note that teamwork and organisation were also highlighted as key to a good learning environment for students. Teamwork is vital when managing various learners' needs in the same clinical setting but also contributes to role modelling safe and effective patient care. A positive teamwork culture has been associated with a decrease in patient mortality within and across a hospital system (Berry et al., 2016) and in addition to role modelling best practice, this culture may reduce students' feelings of conflict and tension which can negatively impact learning (Dale, Leland and Dale, 2013).

b From mentor focus groups

Phase 1: Identification of overarching themes

The mentor focus groups' agreed outputs within their groups were categorised under the development of three themes of management, attributes and coaching.

Table 5.8 Themes from Phase 1 data analysis.

Themes	Examples of data
1 Management *Bureaucratic elements of managing learning*	Time management, organised, action plans, documentation, planning, managing, leadership
2 Attributes *Personal qualities or features of supervisors that influence approach to supporting learning*	Friendly, approachable, supportive, creative, encouraging, empowering, knowledgeable, attentive, calm, adaptive, competent, insightful, experienced, informative, team player, caring, compassionate, patience, empathy, resourceful, adaptive
3 Coaching *Skills to support development of critical thinking, dialogue and leadership*	Open questions, constructive feedback, active listening, feed forward, reflecting, empowering, motivating, evaluate learning, challenge, understands student needs, eye contact, clear objectives, self-awareness, smile, eye contact, engaged, resourceful

Phase 2: Exploration of themes relevant to coaching skills

A higher level of granulation was achieved in the 'attributes' and 'coaching' categories by further sub categorisation of these two themes. The researchers agreed that 'management' referred to a task or approach carried out by mentors and, although important for supporting learning in practice, it was not considered a coaching skill. Therefore, this theme was not further explored.

Table 5.9 Themes from Phase 2 data analysis.

Themes	Sub themes	Examples of data
Attributes	Manner *The first impressions that effect connection with the student*	friendly, approachable, patience, sensitivity, empathy
	Personal ethos *The underlying teaching and learning approach of the mentor*	supportive, encouraging, empowering, creative, motivated, respect
	Expertise *Non-static qualities that were seen as knowledge or profession based*	knowledgeable, good practice, resourceful, adaptive, competent
Coaching	Engaging *Making the initial connection with the learner*	smile, eye contact, good preparation, engaged
	Existing *Establishing learning needs and agreeing goals*	feedback, active listening, self-awareness, open and transparent communication, understanding learning styles and needs of student, empowerment, building confidence
	Expanding *Using coaching skills to enhance learning and develop learners' critical thinking, leadership and decision-making*	reflection, interactive, challenge, problem solving, empowerment, open questioning, feed-forward, constructive feedback, probing questioning, ongoing evaluation of learning, resourceful, comprehensive thinking, interactive, flexible approach

ATTRIBUTES

In a coaching situation, the mentor responses indicated 'attributes' as important to coaching students. These included mentors' underlying professional knowledge and approaches to teaching and learning as well as the manner that mentors displayed to students. This latter point was also supported by the student participants who placed significant value on interpersonal qualities to support learning in practice. Mentors' attitudes, and their manner towards students, have been identified in the literature as pivotal factors which influence positive placement experience as well as students' opinion of their programme as a whole (Dale et al., 2013). Chapter 1 explores comprehensive orientation and socialisation, where the findings show a link between a positive practice learning experience and welcoming characteristics of mentors.

It is recognised that students should have the opportunity to learn in an emotionally safe environment and that a sense of belongingness is a prerequisite for learning in a clinical setting (Levett-Jones and Lathlean, 2008). The mentor's personal ethos to their teaching and support were highlighted as the type of enabling learning identified by Ellstrom (2011).

Interestingly, 'empowerment' was repeatedly highlighted in a number of themes. Empowerment was identified as important to the whole learning process and the ability to be able to negotiate as a professional, with both patients and staff, supports a learning that progresses students to a more challenging and critical standpoint on registration. These are essential differences to the acquiescence that halts any challenge to poor practice identified by Bradbury-Jones, Sambrook and Irvine (2011a, 2011b) and therefore the promotion of learning confidently in practice (Morley, 2015).

Students learnt 'negotiating voice' (Bradbury-Jones et al., 2011b) if they worked in the type of supportive environment researched by Levett-Jones and Lathlean (2009) where students had a sense of 'belongingness' on placement. Where belongingness was not met (Levett-Jones and Lathlean, 2008) students were more likely to be subsumed into the workforce and, through their fear of making mistakes, had no confidence to develop critical thinking. The data analysis from this study suggests that mentor attributes; those of their manner, personal ethos and role modelling of expertise are recognised as important constituents of expansive learning.

COACHING

The coaching theme supports that already identified in 'attributes' and recognises three fundamental areas for supporting students to learn in practice. Initial 'engaging', for example, smiling, eye contact and good preparation with students, came first. Without this professional connection to their supervisor, Morley (2015) found it was difficult for students to settle on placement and progress to active and proactive learning. As well as making this initial connection, mentors also identified the need for supervisors to be able to establish 'existing' students' stage of learning by establishing learning needs and agreeing goals. From this point, the third stage of 'expanding' used coaching skills to enhance established learning and develop learners' critical thinking, leadership and decision-making so it could then be built upon in a socio constructivist manner for student to meet their potential in practice.

Phase 3: Identification of the stages of a coaching model

The themes of 'attributes' and 'coaching' jointly identified a simple and constructivist three stage approach to learning: connecting, establishing and expanding, that is discussed in the conclusion. The initial layers of establishing effective support structures and previous experience was crucial to taking students into an expansive frame of mind for graduate learning.

Conclusion

An 'expansive learning model' (Figure 5.6) was developed from the data analysis of this chapter and demonstrates the progressive coaching steps: connecting, establishing and expanding, that students need to take to achieve higher level critique, reflection and development as a professional. It is based upon a social model of learning that recognises that all members of staff, who the student meets on placement, can play their own and integrated part in students' practice learning. Like the evaluation of CliP (Hill et al., 2015), it recognises the deep investment that is needed in establishing a new coaching model in practice with the demise of the old system of mentorship.

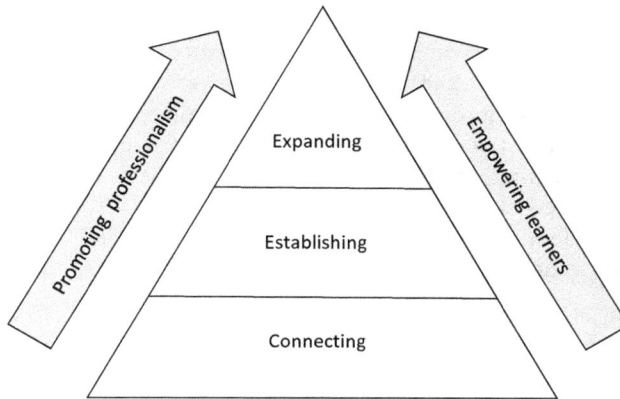

Figure 5.6 Expansive learning model.

The methodology of the use of word clouds to establish widescale opinion in real time with a large group of students proved effective on an engagement level. Students appeared to enjoy the experience of data collection, and its pictorial presentation has since been useful to encourage discussion and debate at mentor events. The wide choice of definition that students used was, however, problematic to gauge specific data and it is recommended that the methodology is used again with the use of agreed terms in order to test the same questions in the future.

The suggested socio-constructivist model of learning that resulted from the research fits well with the organic nature of practice learning (Morley, 2015) and meets the potential of graduates working in a quickly changing environment with a diversity of staff. It provides a mindset for lifelong learning whilst providing a simple coaching model that can be used by all staff in any clinical setting.

The model begins with the 'connecting' stage; an identified, interpersonal connection between the student and their supervisor where mutual engagement and commitment to learning begins. It is evident from the student findings that interpersonal skills, evident in the 'connecting' stage, are key to supporting learning in practice and setting the conditions for achieving expansive learning. Comprehensive orientation and socialisation is further explored in Chapter 1 due its importance and significance to students' learning.

The second stage, 'establishing', is about developing an understanding of the student's current needs and goals and was identified by mentors as listening, providing feedback, communicating and understanding learning styles and needs. In the busyness of practice, both the first and second stage of the model can be forgotten with the risk of eroding students' confidence to progress to expanding their learning on placement (Morley, 2015). With the CLiP model (Hill et al., 2015) it was found that a coach needs to work regularly with the student and any risk to this, including taking a 'hub and spoke' approach, also threatens the first two stages of the model.

The third and final stage, 'expanding', refers to developing the student's critical thinking, critical dialogue, reflexivity and leadership skills. The empowerment of learners, and building professional knowledge, skills and attributes were seen as integral to the whole process and underlined all three stages as a continuum.

The learning culture on placement, and the supervision support within this, are therefore critical factors that determine students' successful learning on placement (Levett-Jones and Lathlean, 2009; Bradbury-Jones et al., 2011a, 2011b). A constraining environment prioritises Ellstrom's (2011) adaptive learning, and it is essential that nursing students learn to appropriately question the nursing care and management they are participating in. Influential to this process is the students' own personality and assertiveness skills which were rarely explored by mentors in their early discussions with student on placement (Morley, 2015). Each stage is irretrievably linked to a holistic coaching model and one that needs to be understood by all staff on placement.

Recommendations

1 Dissemination of the expansive learning model

The model can be piloted and evaluated in a variety of practice learning settings. There is now potential for students and the new roles of supervisors and assessors in both academia and practice to become familiar with the model and explore opportunities to embed it in practice for all learners, at all stages of their learning journey. Any facilitator of students' learning should be supported to simply connect with the student at the beginning of a learning situation, establish the students' level of expertise so learning can be personalised to the students' needs and finally encourage students' questions and self-reflection as a result of their learning.

2 The promotion of dialogic feedback to support expansive learning

The model requires a dialogic approach to feedback to support student empowerment and professional development. Feedback can be formal or informal but should be delivered in a manner that reflects the interpersonal qualities valued by students and where they have an opportunity to question and discuss the feedback being given. The promotion of assessment literacy will enable students to expand their learning beyond what they can achieve as individuals.

Case study for Expansive Learning

The expansive learning chapter identified three levels of learning – connecting, establishing and expanding. This case study highlights how these principles can be used when giving feedback to students.

Sarah is a student nurse who excels in clinical practice. Her practice supervisor/practice assessor wants to encourage Sarah to further reach her potential. She believes that timely discussion with Sarah about her practice will keep Sarah motivated and continuing on a track to 'expand' her learning.

What is the learning aim?

To increase opportunities for dialogic (two-way) feedback for Sarah so future learning is explicit.

What learning will be achieved?

1   To create an environment for feedback where Sarah feels safe and supported to ask questions (connecting).
2   To establish Sarah's prior knowledge and experience before giving feedback (establishing).
3   To link feedback to wider policy (e.g. what does the NMC code say about this?) and alternatives (e.g. if the patient's condition changed how would your nursing care alter?) (expanding).

How can learning be supported?

1 To create an environment for feedback where Sarah feels safe and supported to ask questions (connecting)

Feedback should be encouraged by all members of the team with the emphasis on a coaching style where Sarah is not criticised but encouraged to discuss her nursing care and the underlying rationale. Future experts 'obtain feedback that is accurate, diagnostic and reasonable timely' (Klein, 1998, p. 104). Dialogic feedback is only achieved when students feel confident and safe enough to enter a professional conversation about their performance.

2 To establish Sarah's prior knowledge and experience before giving feedback (establishing)

A constructivist learning theory (Wenger, 1998) argues that building on previous knowledge gives relevance and context to students' learning. '[Learners] enrich their experiences by reviewing prior experiences to derive new insights and lessons from mistakes' (Klein, 1998, p. 104). Encouraging Sarah to reflect on her learning, before feedback is offered, allows her to develop skills to be self-critical of her performance. Sarah should be encouraged to record her feedback in a medium of her choice, so she has a greater opportunity to remember, recall and feedforward her learning.

3 To link feedback to wider policy (e.g. what does the NMC code say about this?) and alternatives (e.g. if the patient's condition changed how would your nursing care alter?) (expanding)

A higher level of performance can exist when registered staff encourage students to reflect on alternative care that could be taken and link their learning to wider policy or nursing theory. Wenger (1998) refers to the first as a strategy of 'imagination' and the second as 'alignment' (Morley, 2016). Encouraging Sarah to expand her learning beyond the immediate can be taken either during individual feedback or in peer learning group. Encouraging Sarah to take responsibility to quiz her peers also sets an early agenda for self-development and peer review.

References

Argyris, C. and Schon, D. (1974) *Theory in practice: Increasing professional effectiveness.* San Francisco, CA: Jossey Bass.
Bazian. (2016) *RCN Mentorship Project 2015: From today's support in practice to tomorrow's vision for excellence.* London: Bazian.
Benner, P. (1984) *From novice to expert: Excellence and power in clinical nursing practice.* Menlo Park, CA: Addison-Wesley Publishing Company.

Berry, J. C., Davis, J. T., Bartman, T., Hafer, C. C., Lieb, L. M., Khan, N. and Brilli, R. J. (2016) 'Improved safety culture and teamwork climate are associated with decreases in patient harm and hospital mortality across a hospital system', *Journal of Patient Safety*. doi:10.1097/PTS.0000000000000251.

Bradbury-Jones, C., Sambrook, S. and Irvine, F. (2011a) 'Empowerment and being valued: A phenomenological study of nursing students' experience of clinical practice', *Nurse Education Today*, 31(5), pp. 368–372.

Bradbury-Jones, C., Sambrook, S. and Irvine, F. (2011b) 'Nursing students and the issue of voice: A qualitative study', *Nurse Education Today*, 31(4), pp. 628–632.

Brown, J. S. and Duguid, P. (1991) 'Organizational learning and communities of practice: Toward a unified view of working, learning and innovation'. *Organization Science*, 2(1), pp. 40–57.

Burns, L. and Gillon, E. (2011) 'Developing an agenda for coaching psychology in undergraduate programmes', *The Coaching Psychologist*, 7(2), pp. 90–97.

Chapman, R. (2001) 'Coping strategies in clinical practice: The nursing students' lived experience', *Contemporary Nurse*, 11(1) p. 95–102

Clarke, D., Williamson, G. R. and Kane, A. (2018) 'Could students' experiences of clinical placements be enhanced by implementing a Collaborative Learning in Practice (CLiP) model?' *Nurse Education in Practice*, 33, pp. A3–A5.

Dale, B., Leland, A. and Dale, J. G. (2013) 'What factors facilitate good learning experiences in clinical studies in nursing: bachelor students' perceptions', *ISRN Nursing*, 2013, pp. 1–8. Available at: https://www.hindawi.com/journals/isrn/2013/628679/ (accessed 11/29/18).

D'Souza, M. S., Karkada, S. N., Parahoo, K. and Venkatesaperumal, R. (2015) 'Perception of and satisfaction with the clinical learning environment among nursing students', *Nurse Education Today*, 35(6), pp. 833–840.

Eccles, S. and Renaud, V. (2018) 'Building students' emotional resilience through placement coaching and mentoring', in Morley, D. A. (ed.) *Enhancing employability in higher education through work based learning*. Switzerland: Palgrave Macmillan, pp. 153–172.

Eden, S. (2014) 'Out of the comfort zone: enhancing work based learning about employability through student reflections on work placement', *Journal of Geography in Higher Education*, 38(2), pp. 266–276.

Ellstrom, P.-E. (2011) 'Informal learning at work: Conditions, processes and logics', in Malloch, M., Cairns, L., Evans, K. & O'Connor, B. (eds.) *The Sage handbook of workplace learning*. London/California/New Delhi/Singapore: Sage Publications Inc., pp. 105–119.

Eraut, M. (2000) 'Non-formal learning and tacit knowledge in professional work', *British Journal of Educational Psychology*, 70(1), pp. 113–136.

Eraut, M. (2004) 'Informal learning in the workplace', *Studies in Continuing Education*, 26(2), pp. 247–273.

Fuller, A. and Unwin, L. (2003) 'Learning as apprentices in the contemporary UK workplace: Creating and managing expansive and restrictive participation', *Journal of Education & Work*, 16(4), pp. 407–426.

Gobbi, M. (2012) 'The hidden curriculum'. Learning the tacit and embodied nature of nursing practice', in Cook, V., Daly, C. & Newman, M. (eds.) *Work-based learning in clinical settings*. London/New York: Radcliffe Publishing, pp. 103–124.

Grant, L. and Kinman, G. (2014) 'Emotional resilience in the helping professions and how it can be enhanced', *Health and Social Care Education*, 3(1), pp. 23–34.

Gray, M. and Smith, L. N. (1999) 'The professional socialization of diploma of higher education in nursing students (Project 2000): a longitudinal study', *Journal of Advanced Nursing*, 29(3), pp. 639–647.

Health Education England (HEE). (2017) 'Case study: Implementing Collaborative Learning in Practice – A new way of learning for nursing students', *Workforce Information Network*. Available at: http://www.ewin.nhs.uk/sites/default/files/eWIN%20Case%20Study%20-%20CLIP%20-%20a%20new%20way%20of%20learning%20for%20student%20nurses.pdf (accessed 06/04/18).

Harteis, C., Morganthaler, B., Kugler, C., Ittner, K.-P., Roth, G. and Graf, B. (2012) 'Professional competence and intuitive decision making: A simulation study in the domain of emergency medicine', *Vocations and Learning*, 5(5), pp. 119–136.

Hill, R., Woodward, M. and Arthur, A. (2015) *Collaborative Learning in Practice (CLiP): Evaluation report*. University of East Anglia, Health Education East of England.

Huggins, D. (2016) 'Enhancing nursing students' education by coaching mentors', *Nursing Management*, 23(1), pp. 30–32.

Klein, G. (1998) *Sources of power: How people make decisions*. Cambridge, MA/London: The MIT Press.

Kuiper, R. A. and Pesut, D. J. (2004) 'Promoting cognitive and metacognitive reflective reasoning skills in nursing practice: Self-regulated learning theory', *Journal of Advanced Nursing*, 45(4), pp. 381–391.

Levett-Jones, T. and Lathlean, J. (2008) 'Belongingness: A prerequisite for nursing students' clinical learning', *Nurse Education Today*, 8(2), pp. 103–111.

Levett-Jones, T. and Lathlean, J. (2009) 'Don't rock the boat: Nursing students' experience of conformity and compliance', *Nurse Education Today*, 29(3), pp. 342–349.

Lobo, C., Arthur, A. and Lattimer, V. (2014) 'Collaborative Learning in Practice (CLiP) for pre-registration nursing students. A background paper for delegates attending the CLiP conference', Collaborative Learning in Practice (CLiP), University of East Anglia, NHS Health Education East of England.

Mackintosh, C. (2006) 'Caring: The socialisation of pre-registration student nurses: A longitudinal qualitative study', *International Journal of Nursing Studies*, 43(8), pp. 953–962.

McIntosh, A., Gidman, J. and Smith, D. (2013) 'Mentors' perceptions and experiences of supporting student nurses in practice', *International Journal of Nursing Practice*, 20(4) pp. 360–365.

Morley, D. A. (2015) 'A grounded theory study exploring first year student nurses' learning in practice', Doctor in Professional Practice thesis. Bournemouth, Bournemouth University.

Morley, D. A. (2016) 'Applying Wenger's communities of practice theory to placement learning', *Nurse Education Today*, 39, pp. 161–162.

Morley, D. A. (2018) 'The "ebb and flow" of student learning on placement', in Morley, D. A. (ed.) *Enhancing employability in higher education through work based learning*. Switzerland: Palgrave Macmillan, pp. 173–190.

Nursing and Midwifery Council (NMC). (2017) *Consultation on standards of proficiency for registered nurses*. Available at: https://www.nmc.org.uk/about-us/consultations/past-consultations/2017-consultations/ (accessed 03/15/19).

Nursing and Midwifery Council (NMC). (2018) 'Guidance on the professional duty of candour'. Available at: https://www.nmc.org.uk/standards/guidance/the-professional-duty-of-candour/ (accessed 11/29/18).

Schon, D. (1983) *The reflective practitioner: How professionals think in action*. Aldershot, UK: Ashgate Publishing Limited.

Spouse, J. (2001) 'Bridging theory and practice in the supervisory relationship: A sociocultural perspective', *Journal of Advanced Nursing*, 33(4), pp. 512–530.

Sundler, A. J., Björk, M., Bisholt, B., Ohlsson, U., Engström, A. K. and Gustafsson, M. (2014) 'Student nurses' experiences of the clinical learning environment in relation to the organisation of supervision: a questionnaire survey', *Nurse Education Today*, 34(4), pp. 661–666.

Wenger, E. (1998) *Communities of practice: Learning, meaning and identity*. New York: Cambridge University Press.

Willis, G. (2015) Raising the bar. Shape of caring: A review of the future education and training of registered nurses and care assistants in England, London. Available at: https://www.hee.nhs.uk/sites/default/files/documents/2348-Shape-of-caring-review-FINAL.pdf (accessed 03/15/19).

6 Future recommendations for practice education: Next steps

Dawn A. Morley (morleydawn@yahoo.co.uk), Kathy Wilson and Natalie Holbery

The strength of practice learning is the authenticity it can bring to the professional development of students, but the positives are counterbalanced by many long recognised challenges of the pedagogy and structures of learning in this environment. 'There is a big difference between a lesson that is about the practice and takes place outside of it, and explanations and stories that are part of the practice and take place within it' (Wenger, 1998, p. 100).

Up to this point, there has been a lack of investment in practice education in the UK (Morley, Wilson and McDermott, 2017) and because of high profile cases of patient neglect (Francis, 2013) and poor student preparation (Willis, 2015) a national response to practice education was initiated. The introduction highlights that, for the time being, the solutions to these challenges have created a vacuum with the removal of the established support structures in practice of students and an increase in new nursing roles, and hence new learners, within the practice setting.

The STEP themes presented in this book have highlighted areas that have potential for development within nursing and midwifery practice education. Unlike many models of clinical practice, it recognises that the clinical environment is unique to each setting with its own variety of resource that can complement the education of students that it supports. 'Like a magpie to the nest, learning is built out of the materials to hand and in relation to the structuring resources of local conditions' (Brown and Duguid, 1991, p. 47).

Practice learning needs to be both accessible and recognisable to students, so it can be used usefully for their development. Evans et al.'s (2010) theory of the recontextualisation of knowledge recognises the difficulty of learning being applicable for students as they move between the university and practice settings. This complexity, and the theory-practice gap that can exist as a result, needs to be addressed and students carefully coached and supported as they negotiate the different learning contexts that are essential to their professional development.

A traditional focus on skills acquisition can, in fact, undermine the need for a more holistic approach to professional development (Eraut, 2004), and this was identified by the student and mentor participants in Chapter 5 on expansive learning. Building students' confidence and self-esteem from the outset is integral to this development and measures such as a comprehensive orientation and socialisation outlined in Chapter 1, and the ability to grow analytical reasoning and empowerment (Bradbury-Jones, Sambrook and Irvine, 2011) through careful use of experienced staff and resources, can support students to meet an appropriate mix of challenge and support (Grealish and Ranse, 2009).

Politically, despite their supernumerary status, students can be subsumed into the workforce and lack of awareness of the structures and pedagogy that support this type of education (Morley, 2015). Eraut (2004) found that novices' work needed to be challenged enough for their level of expertise without it becoming daunting otherwise students develop ineffective coping mechanisms. Appropriate allocation of work and supervision was crucial to promoting students' confidence, so they gain exposure to learning opportunities while simultaneously being supported through the challenging aspects of learning in real life settings. The challenges faced by students in the clinical learning environment has been highlighted in a number of the chapters with the impact of negative learning experiences on student attrition (HEE, 2018) and hence the need to equip them with the skills and confidence to manage these complex environments is paramount.

The social learning theorist Etienne Wenger (1998, p. 268) believes that 'identity is the vehicle that carries our experiences from context to context'. As well as the application of case studies to each chapter, the conclusion brings together the themes to demonstrate how they can be used by students and practitioners. Evans and Rainbird (2006) refer to their concepts for work-based learning as learning *in, for* and *through* the workplace and underlies the importance of integrating and acknowledging the value of practice learning. To draw together the STEP research projects, represented in this book chapters, we will focus here on the cyclical three stages of preparation for practice, practice itself and the transfer of the practice learning back to the academic setting.

1 Preparation for practice

Chapter 1, 'Comprehensive orientation and socialisation', highlights the importance of student preparation before placement (Brown, Stevens and Kermode, 2012) as part of students' long-term socialisation to their future profession (Houghton, 2014). Student participants demonstrated a desire for control over their new learning environment whether it was through additional information or feeling their clinical skills had prepared them better for practice. A peer-led approach, discussed in Chapter 3, highlights a senior student's involvement in preparing junior students for their practice learning experiences and also gave examples of how peers can be used to teach clinical skills prior to placement to the benefit of both 'learner' and 'teacher'. Knowledge and confidence has been strongly linked to empowerment (Bradbury-Jones et al., 2011) and this sets a positive learning culture for students from the beginning of placement.

The book demonstrates that once practice education is viewed as an essential part of the longitudinal socialisation and empowerment to a profession a more pragmatic stance can be taken on how students are prepared for practice beyond a single induction event. A greater emphasis on the promotion of simulation, for example, is evident in new professional guidelines for student nurses (NMC, 2018a).

Preparation for practice learning can be successfully integrated into the university setting by the effective use of resources and prior experience. Part of this process is the wider building of academic-practice partnerships, presented in Chapter 4, where there is a recognition of the importance of understanding the various roles of individuals involved in education and this is of significance with the introduction of the new roles to support supervision and assessment (NMC, 2018c). 'Preparation' is one of the essential themes that arose from the chapter and recommendation were made for organisations to re-examine how they work together in preparing and planning for clinicians and academics to support students in practice. As a result, students can be more comprehensively prepared for learning and working in the very unique environment of real life practice without having to experience the recognised trauma of transition that many students experience (Morley, 2015).

2 Working and learning in practice

Chapter 1 stresses the importance of the induction period of placement as a means of preparing students for the practice learning that follows. Student participants felt that traditional barriers of exclusion could be overcome by a welcoming and structured orientation. Being buddied with a member of the team, with the appropriate attributes to support students during the critical settling in period, was identified as important. Chapter 2, researching the role of 'helpful others' (Eraut, 2007) such as unregistered health care assistants in student clinical education, and Chapter 3 considering the role of student nurse mentors, found both took a significant role in settling students into their placement experience and supporting their learning informally during practice. In both instances the roles were hampered by a lack of understanding and recognition by other placement staff particularly when HCAs and students were used as a back-stop position when registered staff were unavailable.

It was found that the health care assistants role changed as the student matured through their university programme and, as 'helpful others', unregistered staff could play an important role in student development. This was dependent on the appropriate level of supervision and support from registered nurses being in place. The small sample of midwives from Chapter 3 also found the additional support and expertise provided by their student nurse mentors was very helpful to their placement experience. Both chapters recommend a more collaborative, social model of practice learning where students could benefit from a wider breadth of expertise and experience from colleagues in practice.

'Expansive learning', Chapter 5, takes this initial socialisation a stage further and argues for a clinical learning environment that was both enabling (Ellstrom, 2011) and embedded in a social learning model already introduced in Chapter 1. As a result of asking students and mentors about their preferred coaching styles, the chapter presents a simple 'expansive learning' model. This aims to guide any learning facilitator through connecting with the learner, establishing their level of knowledge and expertise before finally supporting students to expand their present learning into the analytical and reflexive professional engagement synonymous with graduate education. This will not be successful without academic-practice partnerships and Chapter 4 highlights the ongoing difficulties of role confusion, accessibility, communication and the lack of joint training opportunities that may impede progress.

Assessment of practice is integral to student learning experience in practice and can at times become the dominate focus for students (Race, 2014). Chapter 4 discusses the importance of ensuring robust and reliable assessment decisions and the need to carefully monitor this with the introduction of the new roles for supervision and assessment outlined by the NMC (2018b). The case study in Chapter 3 highlights the importance of assessment literacy (Price et al., 2012) emphasising the need for students to understand their own assessment requirements to promote their learning and develop as competent practitioners. This understanding can be enhanced through a peer support model where students spend time together exploring each others' views and perceptions to enable them to take more control of their leaning. The case study in Chapter 5 addresses the essential subject of feedback and the importance of constructive feedback with its links to expansive learning. The NMC highlight the importance of constructive feedback to 'promote and encourage reflective learning' as part of student empowerment (NMC, 2018c, p. 11). Carless (2015) highlights the importance of feedback but specifically emphasises student engagement with that feedback and this can be supported when the student returns to the university after a placement experience

3 Learning from the practice experience

Students' experience in practice, when made explicit to them, can be crucial to their understanding of their professional development and the environment in which they have been both learning and working. By working with, and being supported by, unregistered staff and peer students on placement, student participants in Chapters 1 and 2 began to challenge traditional hierarchal roles in practice and value the collaborative effort of genuine team working. Chapter 4 promoted this further by encouraging placement areas to take a systematic and focused approach to student support that could be inclusive of all staff in the practice setting and outlines how the various roles proposed by the NMC (NMC, 2018b) could work together to support the student learning and assessment in practice in the case studies.

The introduction of these new professional roles of practice supervisor, practice assessor and academic assessor (NMC, 2018b), as part of the revised model for practice learning, presents us with an excellent opportunity to improve the overall student experience and outcomes. This, however, requires significant investment and support to change the current culture and manage these changes in a healthcare system that is understaffed (CoDH, 2016).

Critically, student practice learning needs to be brought back into the academic setting for analysis and reflection so that students' experience is used effectively going forward. Evans et al. (2010) discuss the 'gradual release' of sequential elements of the curriculum whereby theoretical knowledge is developed alongside students' practice skills. In this circumstance, the gradual release occurs when practice is further linked back to theory post placement as a foundation for building students' ongoing professional education. Winstone and Avery (2018) researched the potential of the transfer of 'practice to theory' when psychology students used their work-based learning in the academic curriculum that followed. Their results demonstrated the value of using this approach as students were able to interpret new course content from a more advanced practice perspective.

Overall, the book has taken known areas of friction within practice learning and has scrutinised these further through five separate research projects. The research teams were supported through the HEE funded STEP project and through this process developed recommendations for further practice development for student nurses and midwives. The need for the education of the future workforce to keep up with the pace of changes in healthcare delivery has been recognised in many reports (Willis, 2015; CoDH, 2016) and at a time of great change in professional practice education the authors hope that their chapters will instil a sense of empowerment and alternative thinking in approaches to practice learning.

References

Bradbury-Jones, C., Sambrook, S. and Irvine, F. (2011) 'Empowerment and being valued: A phenomenological study of nursing students' experience of clinical practice', *Nurse Education Today*, 31(4), pp. 368–372.

Brown, J. S. and Duguid, P. (1991) 'Organizational learning and communities of practice: Toward a unified view of working, learning and innovation', *Organization Science*, 2(1), pp. 40–57.

Brown, J., Stevens, J., and Kermode, S. (2012) 'Measuring student nurse professional socialisation: The development and implementation of a new instrument', *Nurse Education Today*, 33(6), pp. 565–573.

Carless, D., (2015) *Excellence in university assessment: Learning from award-winning practice.* London: Routledge.

Council of Deans of Health (CoDH). (2016) 'Educating the future nurse – A paper for discussion'. Available at: https://councilofdeans.org.uk/wp-content/uploads/2016/08/Educating-the-Future-Nurse-FINAL-1.pdf (accessed 10/15/18).

Ellstrom, P.-E. (2011) 'Informal learning at work: Conditions, processes and logics' in Malloch, M., Cairns, L., Evans, K. & O'Connor, B. (eds.) *The Sage handbook of workplace learning.* London/ California/New Delhi/Singapore: Sage Publication Inc., pp. 105–119.

Eraut, M. (2004) 'Informal learning in the workplace', *Studies in Continuing Education*, 26(2), pp. 247–273.

Eraut, M. (2007) 'Learning from other people in the workplace', *Oxford Review of Education*, 33(4), pp. 403–422.

Evans, K. and Rainbird, H. (2006) 'Workplace learning: Perspectives and challenges' in Evans, K., Hodkinson, P., Rainbird, H. & Unwin, L. (eds.) *Improving workplace learning.* London: Routledge.

Evans, K., Guile, D., Harris, J. and Allan, H. (2010) 'Putting knowledge to work: A new approach', *Nurse Education Today*, 30(3), pp. 245–251.

Francis, R. (2013) *Report of the Mid Staffordshire NHS Foundation Trust public inquiry. Volume 1: Analysis of evidence and lessons learned (part 1).* HC 898- I. London: The Stationery Office.

Grealish, L. and Ranse, K. (2009) 'An exploratory study of first year nursing students' learning in the clinical workplace', *Contemporary Nurse*, 33(1), pp. 80–92.

Health Education England (HEE). (2017) 'Case study: Implementing Collaborative Learning in Practice – A new way of learning for nursing students', *Workforce Information Network*. Available at: http://www.ewin.nhs.uk/sites/default/files/eWIN%20Case%20Study%20-%20CLIP%20-%20a%20new%20way%20of%20learning%20for%20student%20nurses.pdf (accessed 11/02/18).

Houghton, C. E. (2014) '"Newcomer adaptation": A lens through which to understand how nursing students fit in with the real world of practice', *Journal of Clinical Nursing*, 23(15–16) pp. 2367–2375.

Morley, D. A. (2015) 'A grounded theory study exploring first year student nurses' learning in practice', Doctor in Professional Practice thesis. Bournemouth, Bournemouth University.

Morley, D. A., Wilson, K. and McDermott, J. (2017) 'Changing the practice learning landscape', *Nurse Education in Practice*, 27, pp. 169–171.

Nursing and Midwifery Council (NMC). (2018a) *Realising professionalism: Standards for education and training. Part 3: Standards for pre-registration nursing programmes.* United Kingdom: Nursing & Midwifery Council.

Nursing and Midwifery Council (NMC). (2018b) *Realising professionalism: Standards for education and training. Part 1: Standards framework for nursing and midwifery education.* United Kingdom: Nursing & Midwifery Council.

Nursing and Midwifery Council (NMC). (2018c) *Realising professionalism: Standards for education and training. Part 2: Standards for student supervision and assessment.* United Kingdom: Nursing & Midwifery Council.

Price, M., Rust, C., O'Donovan, B.Handley, K. and Bryant, R. (2012) *Assessment literacy: The foundation for improving student learning.* Assessment Standards Knowledge exchange (ASKe). Oxford: Oxford Brooks University.

Race, P. (2014) *Making learning happen: A guide for post-compulsory education.* Third edition. London/ California/New Delhi/Singapore: Sage Publications Ltd.

Wenger, E. (1998) *Communities of practice: Learning, meaning and identity.* New York: Cambridge University Press.

Willis, G. (2015) Raising the bar. Shape of caring: A review of the future education and training of registered nurses and care assistants in England, London. Available at: https://www.hee.nhs.uk/sites/default/files/documents/2348-Shape-of-caring-review-FINAL.pdf (accessed 03/15/19).

Winstone, N. and Avery, R. (2018) 'Enhancing psychology students' employability through 'practice to theory' learning following a professional training year' in Morley, D. (ed.) *Enhancing employability in higher education through work-based learning.* Switzerland: Palgrave Macmillan, pp. 213–233.

Index

Page numbers in *italics* indicate illustrations, **bold** a table

For Product Safety Concerns and Information please contact our EU
representative GPSR@taylorandfrancis.com
Taylor & Francis Verlag GmbH, Kaufingerstraße 24, 80331 München, Germany

www.ingramcontent.com/pod-product-compliance
Lightning Source LLC
Chambersburg PA
CBHW081110220326
41598CB00038B/7303